AF332917

PEANUT ALLERGIES

SYMPTOMS, MANAGEMENT AND PREVENTION

Immunology and Immune System Disorders

IMMUNOLOGY AND IMMUNE SYSTEM DISORDERS

PEANUT ALLERGIES

SYMPTOMS, MANAGEMENT AND PREVENTION

MARIA PELE, PhD

AND

CARMEN CIMPEANU, PhD

EDITORS

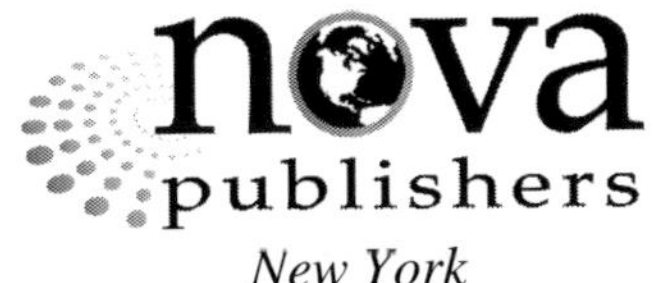

nova publishers

New York

NOTICE TO THE READER

Library of Congress Cataloging-in-Publication Data

ISBN: 978-1-63484-742-1
Library of Congress Control Number: 2016932151

Published by Nova Science Publishers, Inc. † New York

CONTENTS

PREFACE

Food allergies have a considerable impact on modern society. Some of the most severe allergic reactions occur when peanuts and peanut derivatives are consumed. The main causative agents of a peanut allergy are proteins. The total protein content of a peanut is represented by thirty-two different proteins, of which about eighteen (nearly 7-10%) have been identified as capable of binding specific IgE, and so can be considered allergenic. Comprised of six chapters, this book comprehensively covers all topics of peanut allergy. A unique, concise and up-to-date resource, it offers readers an innovative and valuable presentation of the subject. It has been carefully prepared to present the concepts with the help of diagrams and tables. Each chapter is presented in a simple and systematic way to provide a thorough understanding of the core aspects of peanut allergy and the components of peanuts which cause allergic reactions. The basic concepts of clinical aspects, peanut allergens properties, cross reactivity and stability of peanut allergens and the legislation to protect sensitive people are clearly explained. Recent discoveries of peanut allergens are highlighted. From the description of the first peanut allergen called Ara h1 in 1991, so far there have been about thirteen proteins with allergenic action described. The allergenic proteins in a peanut, named Ara h1 – Ara h17 and agglutinin have been identified, largely characterized and accepted by the Allergen Nomenclature Subcommittee of the International Union of Immunological Societies (IUIS). Some of these allergens have established structural features, biochemical and physicochemical properties and their biosynthesis genes encoded. Being proteins, peanut allergens can suffer some modifications during food processing and digestion (acylation, polymerization, nitration, Maillard reaction etc.), and interactions within complex food matrices (both natural and fabricated structures). These modifications can reduce or increase their allergenic properties and are influenced by the food matrix. Peanut allergens have different cross-reactions with other allergens such as, for example, those of soybean, peas, lima beans, green beans, chickpeas, lentils or other beans. Methods commonly used to detect and quantify peanut allergens are mainly immunochemical and molecular methods. However, methods have been developed based on HPLC techniques coupled both with and without mass spectrometry, capillary electrophoresis, circular dichroism, FTIR or NMR. Peanut allergy is high and there is currently no treatment for it. There is a lethal risk associated with peanut allergy, and in order to protect public health, the regulatory bodies worldwide will issue legislation concerning a requirement to clearly have a warning label of the possible presence of food allergens. The last chapter contains some of the most used preventive actions and elaborated legislation in different countries.

In: Peanut Allergies
Editors: M. Pele and C. Cimpeanu

ISBN: 978-1-63484-742-1
© 2016 Nova Science Publishers, Inc.

INTRODUCTION:
PEANUT ALLERGIES

Carmen Cimpeanu, PhD[*]
University of Agronomic Sciences and Veterinary Medicine,
Bucharest, Romania

ABSTRACT

Peanuts history began over 7,000 years ago. Their origin is in South America from where were spread worldwide. Nowadays, practically peanuts are consummated in the countries of the whole world, indifferent forms. This fact is due to the exceptional nutritional value of this legume. However along with the nutritive value, peanuts have determined, especially in developed countries, the development of a disease, namely peanut allergy. Unfortunately, it seems that prevalence of this disease increases every year. Because there is still no cure for this disease are required detailed knowledge of the allergy itself, the nature of the substances that cause the disease, the ways to identify these substances in various matrices and finally the development of suitable treatments.

Keywords: history, peanut quality, peanut allergy

---

[*] Corresponding Author address. Email: carmencimpeanu@yahoo.com.

INTRODUCTION

The peanut, known also as groundnut, goober peas, earthnuts, pignuts or pygmy nuts (Latin name *Arachis hypogaea*), is a food that nowadays, is practically part from the alimentation of the worldwide population.

Anthropologists have found evidence of peanut cultivation dating back at least 7,600 years in South America, in Peru and Bolivia. However, it seems that the early domestication of peanut cultivation has taken place in Paraguayan valleys. In pre-Columbian culture, peanuts occupied a place of honor, being found in various art forms such as sculpture and jewelry, used in sacrificial offerings and entombed them with mummies, making an intoxicating beverage together with maize for celebrations, as well serving as money [1]. The peanuts spread in Mexico by the 1st century AC.

It must be mentioned that, recent archeological discoveries provide evidences of the presence of peanut seeds during the Neolithic period in China (around 4000 BC). Although, no written documents mentioning peanut cultivation in this period in China have been discovered [2]. After the discovery of America by Christopher Columbus in 1492, colonization of South Central and North America and the formation of new states throughout a period of about 300 years, the colonists have contributed to spread peanut plants worldwide. Thus, by the 1500s the Portuguese transplanted peanuts to West Africa, the Spaniards introduced them to the Philippines and sailors transported to China too [3]. The peanut plant was mainly a garden crop during the colonial period in North America. Africans were the first people to introduce peanuts to North America beginning in the 1700s as part of the slave trade and were considered an inferior status and where it was used mostly as food for the poor and livestock.

Peanuts became prominent after the Civil War because both Armies subsisted on this nutritious protein source. With the development of the industrial revolution from the 19th century, early 20th century equipment was invented for planting, cultivating, harvesting and picking peanuts from the plants, as well as for shelling and cleaning the kernels. With these significant mechanical aids, demand for peanuts grew rapidly, especially for oil, roasted and salted nuts, peanut butter and candy. In this context, in the early 1900s peanuts became a significant agricultural crop. In this period, renewed scientist Dr. George Washington Carver promoted crop rotation practices and the cultivation of peanuts. Furthermore, he developed more than 300 uses for peanuts from recipes to new products and even non-food uses.

Due to its nutritional qualities, peanuts have become an integral part of soldiers' alimentation during the two wars and also in confectionary industry after Second World War [4, 5].

Nowadays, peanuts enjoy a widespread and worldwide use thanks to its special qualities. Peanut is a legume but between vegetables and nuts, peanuts contains a bigger amount of protein (20-26%), 40-50% oil and a lot of valuable nutrients such as antioxidants, vitamins, minerals and coenzymes like Coenzyme Q10. It is important to mention that contrary to other legumes peanuts contains all the essential amino acids necessary for normal body growth and metabolism [6]. Peanuts are consumed in many forms such as boiled peanuts, peanut oil, peanut butter, roasted peanuts, and added peanut meal in snack food, energy bars, candies, spicy sauce or meat dishes. It can be used for garden bird feeding and as protein cake is used as animal feed. In addition, peanuts can be used in different industrial end uses like paint, varnish, lubricating oil, leather dressings, furniture polish, insecticides, nitro-glycerine, soap, cosmetics, some textile fibres, wallboard, abrasives, fuel, glue and others. The top three producers of peanuts in the world are China, India and USA. In a statistics of 6 years average (2009 – 2014) peanut production inshell basis, producers order by percentage is: China – 41%, India – 15%, USA – 6%, Nigeria – 6%, Indonesia – 3%, Argentina – 3% Vietnam – 1% and others – 25% [7]. Yet even if, China ranks listed as producer, the major exporters are USA, Argentina, Sudan, Senegal and Brazil. The major peanut importers are European Union, Canada and Japan. The European Union is the largest consuming region in the world that does not produce peanuts. Thus, in Europe, about 550.000 MT of peanuts are consumed each year. Almost all of its consumption is supplied by imports (99%). Consumption of peanuts in the EU is primarily as food, mostly as roasted-in-shell peanuts and as shelled peanuts used in confectionery and bakery products [8].

Although many people enjoy foods made with peanuts, there are pretty much the people who have mild to severe peanut allergy reactions. The term "allergy" was introduced in 1906 by Clemens P. Pirquet to describe both protective immunity and hypersensitivity reactions [9]. Over time the term is used for adverse reactions to an irritant that the body perceives as harmful. The allergy symptoms are wide and depend of patient from varying degrees of drippy, stuffy, achy nose, crusty or itchy until the worst, death.

Peanut allergens are the most hazardous food allergens, especially in European Union, United State of America and Australia.

The prevalence of peanut allergy among children in Western countries has increased in the last 10 – 15 years, and peanut allergy is becoming apparent in

Africa (Ghana) and Asia [10, 11]. It seems that nearly 100,000 new cases annually, affect some 1 in 50 primary school-aged children in the United States, Canada, the United Kingdom, and Australia [11]. So, at least 2% adults and 6-8% children have peanut allergy [11 - 18].

Peanut is the most allergenic food with no treatment no disappearance in outgrown and sometimes with fatal consequences. In addition, peanut allergens have different cross-reactions with other allergens such as, for example, those of soybean, peas, lima beans, green beans, chickpeas, lentils or other beans. Being proteins, peanut allergens can suffer some modifications during food processing and digestion (acylation, polymerization, nitration, Maillard reaction etc.), interactions within complex food matrices (both natural and fabricated structures). There is currently no treatment for peanut allergy, so all these aspects increase threats to susceptible individuals.

To protect those people who have food allergies and to protect health of citizens, at least developer countries established legislation which mandates clear labelling of specific food allergens.

CONCLUSION

Peanuts are some of the most complex foods, being rich in nutrients needed for normal body growth and metabolism. Although only in the 20th century began to be widely produced, only now it has become a food consumed all over the world in various forms. Despite of extension peanut allergy, even in countries in Asia, epidemiological data are still needed, especially in developing countries where in the last decades, this phenomenon has grown. There are many aspects of peanut allergy who are not yet clearly known, for example, what causes this disease whose prevalence has increased so much. Depth studies are needed to establish a treatment which to remove at least the prospect of a fatal case. At this point it is necessary that the laws established by each country, by allergy associations worldwide, by the World Allergy Organization to be strictly followed.

REFERENCES

[1]   Dillehay, T.D., (2007). Earliest-known evidence of peanut, cotton and squash farming found. http://www.eurekalert.org/pub_releases/2007-06/vu-eeo062507.php.

[2]   Yao, G., (2004). Peanut Production and Utilization in the People's Republic of China, University of Georgia, http://www.lanra.uga.edu/peanut/download/china.pdf

[3]   Krause, S., Latendorf, T., Schmidt, H., Darcan-Nicolaisen, Y., Reese, G., Petersen, A., Janssen, O., Becker, W-M., (2010). Peanut varieties with reduced Ara h 1 content indicating no reduced allergenicity. *Mol. Nutr. Food Res. 54*, 381–387

[4]   World Geography of the Peanut. University of Georgia. http://web.archive.org/web/20060901131608/http://www.lanra.uga.edu/peanut/knowledgebase/

[5]   Putnam, D.H., Oplinger, E.S., Teynor, T.M., Oelke, E.A., Kelling, K.A., and Doll, J.D., (2013). Alternative field crops manual – Peanut. Purdue University. https://www.hort.purdue.edu/newcrop/afcm/peanut.html

[6]   Settaluri, V.S., Kandala, C.V.K., Puppala, N., Sundaram, J., (2012). Peanuts and their Nutritional Aspects—A Review. *Food and Nutrition Sciences. 3*, 1644-1650.

[7]   INC, International Nut & Dried Fruit, Global Statistical Review 2014-2015.

[8]   European Nut Association, http://www.groundnuts.eu/europe

[9]   Silverstein, A., (2000). Clemens Freiherr von Pirquet: Explaining immune complex disease in 1906. *Nat. Immunol.,* 1(6), 453-455.

[10]   Du Toit, G., Roberts, G., Sayre, P.H., Bahnson, H.T., Radulovic, S., Santos, A.F., M.D., Brough, H.A., Phippard, D., Basting, M., Feeney, M., Victor Turcanu, V., Sever, M.L., Gomez Lorenzo, Plaut, M., Lack, G., (2015). Randomized Trial of Peanut Consumption in Infants at Risk for Peanut Allergy. *N Engl J Med,* 372, 803-813.

[11]   Fleischer, D.M., Sicherer, S., Greenhawt, M., Campbell, D., Chan, E.S., Muraro, A., Halken, S., Katz, Y., Ebisawa, M., Eichenfield, L., Sampson, H., for the LEAP Trial Team and Secondary Contributors. (2015). Consensus communication on early peanut introduction and the prevention of peanut allergy in high-risk infants. *Allergy, Asthma, and Clinical Immunology: Official Journal of the Canadian Society of Allergy and Clinical Immunology, 11*(1), 23.

[12] Woods, R.K., Abramson, M., Bailey, M., Walters, E.H., (2001). International prevalences of reported food allergies and intolerances. Comparisons arising from the European Community Respiratory Health Survey (ECRHS) 1991-1994. *Eur J Clin Nutr* 55(4), 298-304.

[13] Al-Muhsen, S., Clarke, A.E., Kagan, R.S., (2003). Peanut allergy: an overview. *CMAJ,* 168(10), 1279-1285.

[14] Hourihane, J. O., Knulst, A.C., (2005). Thresholds of allergenic proteins in foods. *Toxicol. Appl. Pharm.*, 207, S152 - S156.

[15] Sicherer, S.H., Muñoz-Furlong, A., Godbold, J.H., Sampson, H.A., (2010). US prevalence of self-reorted peanut, tree nut, and sesame allergy: 11-year follow-up. *J Allergy Clin Immunol*;125, 1322-1326.

[16] Soller, L., Ben-Shoshan, M., Harrington, D.W., Fragapane, J., Joseph, L., St Pierre, Y., Godefroy, S.B., La Vieille, S., Elliot, S.J., Clarke, A.E., (2012). Overall prevalence of self-reported food allergy in Canada. *J Allergy Clin Immunol*. 130, 986-988.

[17] Amoah, A.S., Obeng, B.B., Larbi, I.A., Versteeg, S.A., Aryeetey, Y., Akkerdaas, J.H., Zuidmeer, L., Lidholm, J., Fernandez-Rivas, M., Hartgers, F.C., Boakye, D.A., van Ree, R., Yazdanbakhsh, M., (2013). Peanut-specific IgE antibodies in asymptomatic Ghanaian children possibly caused by carbohydrate determinant cross-reactivity. *J Allergy Clin Immunol* 132, 639-647.

[18] Nwaru, B.I., Hickstein, L., Panesar, S.S., Muraro, A., Werfel, T., Cardona, V, Dubois, A,E.J., Halken, S., Hoffmann-Sommergruber, K., Poulsen, L.K., Roberts, G., van Ree, R., Vlieg-Boerstra, B.J., Sheikh, A., on behalf of the EAACI Food Allergy and Anaphylaxis Guidelines Group, (2014). The epidemiology of food allergy in Europe: a systematic review and meta-analysis. *Allergy,* 69, 62–75.

In: Peanut Allergies
Editors: M. Pele and C. Cimpeanu

ISBN: 978-1-63484-742-1
© 2016 Nova Science Publishers, Inc.

Chapter 1

SYMPTOMS, MANAGEMENT AND THERAPY

Diana Deleanu, PhD
University of Medicine and Pharmacy Iuliu Hatieganu,
Allergy Department, Cluj-Napoca, Romania

ABSTRACT

Food allergies may affect 2-8% of the children and 1-2% of the adult population. A few number of foods, 8-14 foods, produce 90-95% of the symptoms of food allergy, peanut being one of the most frequent allergen inducing severe symptoms. The prevalence of peanut allergy is 0.6% in USA and is also increasing in West Europe. Peanut allergy is a long lasting allergy (usually children do not out grow their peanut allergy). The symptoms of peanut allergy are induced by 2-3 allergen contained in peanuts (Arah1, Ara h2 and Ara h6). Symptoms are mediated by specific IgE and are urticaria, itch, angioedema, eczema, asthma, gastro-intestinal manifestations, anaphylaxis. Some of the allergic patients died due to severe anaphylaxis. Diagnosis of peanut allergy is based on specific IgE evaluation (skin prick tests, serum evaluation), food challenge. Management of the peanut allergy is avoidance and therapy of the manifestation. Patients should be educated to avoid peanut in different foods, to have their emergency kit, including auto-administrated epinephrine. In the last years different trials have succeeded of inducing tolerance to peanut by oral immunotherapy. To prevent to development of peanut allergy it is recommended to introduce peanuts early in life, as LEAP study demonstrated.

Keywords: peanuts, anaphylaxis, oral immunotherapy

INTRODUCTION

Peanut allergy is one of the most common food allergy [1, 2, 3]. It is thought to is the most common food allergy in infants [3, 4]. Adults prevalence of peanut allergy is not known, but a population survey found that 0.6% of the US population and 0.5% of the British population believe to have peanut allergy [1]. Fatal reactions [5] to peanuts confirm the importance of peanuts in the etiology of food allergies.

Definition. Peanut allergy is one of the most causes of severe allergy attacks with life-threatening symptoms, even to tiny amounts of peanut.

History. First cases of peanut allergy were reported in 70' with an epidemic increase in the late 80' and 90'. First cases of food-induced anaphylaxis were published in 1988 [6] and in 90% of the fatalities, peanuts and nuts are the allergens [7]. There are arguments that the use of peanut oil skin (called also arachis oil) in young children might be a possible factor for the increase in peanut allergy [8]. In a cohort study, 49 children with history of peanut allergy (peanut allergy was confirmed by peanut challenge in 23 children out of 36) the analysis of interview data showed a significant independent relation of peanut allergy with the use of skin preparations containing peanut oil (odds ratio, 6.8; 95% confidence interval, 1.4 to 32.9) (Table 1). The current opinion does not support this theory [9] and in the the European Commission report on peanut oil published in 2014 it is shown that a much lower quantity of peanut allergen penetrates the skin, not enough to sensitized (Table 1).

Epidemiology. Peanut allergy is one that frequently results in anaphylaxis. The highest prevalence of peanut allergy is in United States. Telephone surveys, conducted from 1997 to 2008 evaluated self-reported peanut allergy to 0.6% in children and 1.6% in adults [11, 12, 13]. The prevalence of peanut allergy is increasing in the last years in children (up to 2.1%), but not in adults [11, 12]. The prevalence of peanut allergy is also increasing in Europe, but is lower in some other countries. In UK, the prevalence of peanut allergy in children is 1.85%, much higher than in Israel (0.17%) [14]. The difference is correlated to the early consumption of peanut in Israeli children.

This allergy is rarely outgrow; only less than 20% of the allergic patients reported a tolerance later to peanut. In a study only 9.6% of the allergic children could had a negative challenge upon a median 5-years follow-up [15].

Exposure to peanuts can occur in various ways direct, cross-contact or inhalation. Direct contact is the most frequent contact with the peanut allergen is eating peanuts or peanut-containing foods. Sometimes direct skin contact with peanuts (peanut oil in cosmetics) can trigger an allergic reaction. It is assume that this penetration of peanuts occur in the 50'-60' to induce the epidemics of peanut allergy. Across-contact is the unintended introduction of peanuts into a product. It's generally the result of a food being exposed to peanuts during processing or handling. The third way to be expose to peanuts is inhalation. An allergic reaction may occur when the dust or aerosols containing peanuts are inhaled. It can happen from a source such as peanut flour or peanut oil cooking spray.

Table 1. Relation of peanut oil skin preparations and peanut allergy [8]

Use of peanut- oil preparations	Peanut Allergy		Positive Peanut Challenge	
	Unadjusted OR (95% CI)	Adjusted OR (95% CI)*	Unadjusted OR (95% CI)	Adjusted OR (95% CI)*
Yes	7.49 (1,71-32.8)	6.81 (1.41-32.9)	9.00 (1.15-70.4)	8.34 (1.05-66.1)
No	1.00	1.00	1.00	1.00
P value	0.008	0.02	0.04	0.045
One time-skin whole body application of peanut-oil with 0.5 ppm**			10 microgram peanut allergen (lower than the 200 microgram needed for save challenges) !!!	

OR denotes odds ratio, and CI confidence interval. Children who did not use the creams served as the reference group. *Odds ratio have been adjusted for the consumption of soy milk or soy formula; rash over joints and in skin crease; and oozing, crusted rash. ** European Commission. Scientific Committee on Consumer Safety [9].

SYMPTOMS

An allergic response to peanuts usually occurs within minutes (!) after exposure (5-30 minutes). One peanut contains 200 mg of protein, an allergic may react to even traces (100 µg) of peanut (less than 1 peanut) [2]. The average age of onset of the symptoms for peanut allergy is 18 months.

Peanut allergy signs and symptoms can affect skin, respiratory, gastrointestinal system and most severe are systemic with cardiovascular involvement (Table 2).

Skin. Skin reactions are hives (Figure 1), itch, redness, swelling (angioedema). Itching may occur all over the body or around the mouth (Figure 2) and throat (that may be a sign of severe manifestation – angioedema of the larynx). Angioedema of the larynx may be life-threatening due to respiratory failure. In some children, peanut consumption may aggravate the atopic dermatitis. Sometimes a flare eczema may develop [10].

Respiratory symptoms. Patients may develop runny nose, itch, shortness of the breath or even wheeze, Asthmatic patients are at risk.

Gastro-intestinal manifestation may include stomach cramps, nausea, vomiting, diarrhea.

Systemic manifestation are hypotension and anaphylactic shock. Fatal anaphylaxis may develop. The prevalence of anaphylaxis is difficult to be estimated; a Danish study found 20 cases of anaphylactic shock outside hospital with 3.2 cases per 100.000 inhabitants per year, 5% were fatal [16]. In Mayo Clinic Emergency department over 3.5 years period, foods were the most frequent cause of anaphylaxis: 59 cases of 142 with identified allergen [17]. Bock concluded that in US at least 950 cases of severe food-induced anaphylaxis occur each year, peanuts and nuts being the most common cause [18].

**Table 2. Frequency of target system involvement in first presentation
of peanut allergy [2, 10]**

Target system	% of patients
Cutaneous	
Urticaria, erythema, angioedema	83 – 89
Flashing Eczema	11
Respiratory	
Wheezing, stridor, cough, dyspnea, throat tightness, nasal congestion	7 – 42
Gastrointestinal	26
Vomiting, diarrhea, abdominal pain	13
Cardiovascular Hypotension, arrhythmia, cardiac arrest	4

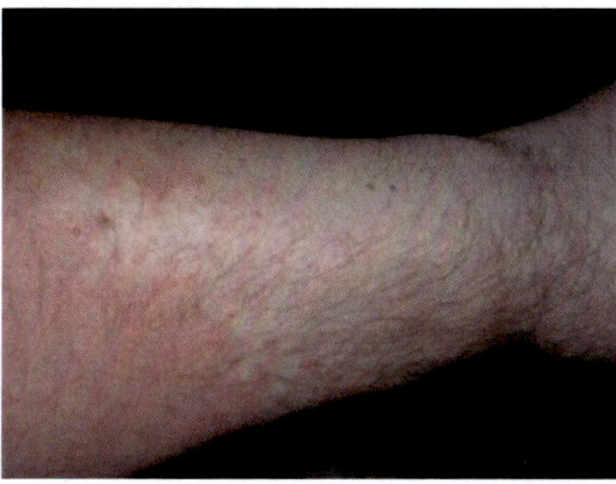

Figure 1. Hives in a peanut allergic patient.

In anaphylaxis skin, upper and lower airways, gastrointestinal, neurologic and cardiovascular sign and symptoms may develop and their onset is variable. The most common sign of anaphylaxis is urticaria and angioedema, occurring in 80-90% of the patients. They may be associated with flushing and generalized itch. In 60% of the patients airways are involved with shortness of breath, dyspnea and wheeze. Laryngeal edema, or edema of tongue, lips may be present. Dysphagia and dysphonia can be present. Almost 50% of the patients develop hypotension. Death is due to anaphylaxis either severe hypotension (shock), either to respiratory obstruction (laryngeal edema).

Some other symptoms may be uterine and bladder cramps.

The symptoms may develop between 5-30 minutes after ingestion, the more rapid is the onset, the more severe is the anaphylactic shock. Probably, peanuts are the most common cause of death due to food anaphylaxis in United States [19]. The majority of the patients may recover either spontaneously or after treatment (adrenaline/epinephrine administration).

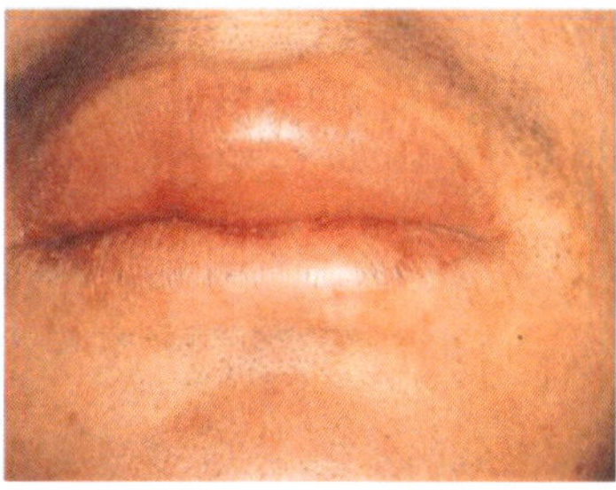

Figure 2. Angioedema of the lips in a peanut allergic patient.

Some anaphylactic reaction are biphasic in nature, with an early phase (5-30 minutes) and a late phase follows after 1-8 hours. Sometimes the symptoms of anaphylaxis may be protected and can last continuously for 5-32 hours [20].

Mild symptoms can last up to an hour but severe symptoms can last longer and the anaphylactic shock may be biphasic or protected.

Some people with peanut allergy might also react to some vegetables (legumes) like soya, green beans, kidney beans, baked beans and green peas because these foods contain similar allergens to peanuts.

DIAGNOSTIC

Diagnosing a peanut allergy can be complicated. Symptoms can vary from person to person, and a single individual may not always experience the same symptoms during every reaction.

It is very important to have a food diary before to point any reactions. The dairy should contain what (and how much) was ate; when the symptoms started (timing), how long did they bothered (duration of the symptoms), what did alleviated them. Also different circumstances should be noted (e.g., exercise).

For the diagnostic is necessary to evaluate the presence of specific IgE to peanut allergens. That can be evaluated by skin prick tests or from serum.

In Vivo Tests

Skin prick tests are performed on forearm or on the back. They are read at 15–30 minutes. Antihistamines should not be taken before the skin prick tests at least 3 days (their consumption can block the allergic reaction and is seen on histamine control).

Commercial extracts (rarely raw material) are used. A positive reaction is greater than 3 mm wheal or more than negative saline control, at least half of histamine (positive control). There are cut off levels for the skin prick test which give a high positive predictive value for the test. If the diameter of wheal is higher than 14 mm, it is considered that the challenge test is not needed anymore.

In Vitro **Tests**

The blood test will find the presence of specific IgE to peanuts using radioallergosorbent (RAST) tests or an enzyme-linked immune assay (ELISA) tests or CAP-System FEIA (have the highest sensitivity and specificity). IgE specific to major allergens (ARA h1, Ara h2, and Ara h3) are used in commercial kits. Normal values are lower than 0.35 kUA/L. There is a high correlation between skin prick tests and serum level of specific IgE to peanuts (Table 3). IgE specific higher than15kUIA/L has a high specificity for allergy to peanuts and there is no need for a food challenge for diagnostic (in symptomatic patients).

Specific IgE (both skin prick test and serum) may be positive without any symptoms in half of the patients. For a diagnostic is necessary to do food challenge. Negative specific IgE to peanuts exclude allergy (negative predictive value 100%) (Table 3).

Other test are not so relevant for food-induced anaphylaxis, so the evaluation of tryptase do not increase significantly [16]. Histamine levels increase in the first minutes and remains elevated for a brief period of time after the allergic reaction.

FOOD CHALLENGE

Because a peanut allergy can be difficult to diagnose through skin tests or blood tests, it is a good idea to introduce a peanut elimination diet, in which any peanut or peanut-product to be avoided for a specific period of time (two to four weeks). If your symptoms improve when the item is removed from the diet, it's likely that you the patient is allergic to peanuts.

If the food elimination diet produces inconclusive results, your allergist may recommend an oral food challenge.

The gold standard for food allergy is double-blind placebo-controlled food challenge (DBPLFC). Peanuts should be eliminated DBPCFC for 10-14 days and also antihistamines should be discontinued [19]. The DBPCFO is performed in the specialized allergy hospitals because there is a risk to develop a severe reaction in very sensitive patients. During this test, the patient is fed with tiny amounts of peanut or peanut-based products or placebo (with the same taste, smell) in double-blind placebo-controlled manner. The dose is usually double every 30-60 minutes. Over a period of time, the dose is increased and any sign or symptoms are noted. Patients with anaphylactic shock should not be challenged!

Emergency medication and emergency equipment will be on hand during this procedure in case of a severe reaction.

An algorithm for the peanut allergy is illustrated in Figure 3.

**Table 3. Performance characteristics of diagnostic tests
for peanut allergy [2, 10]**

Diagnostic test	Sensitivity	Specificity	Positive, predictive value	Positive, predictive value
	%	%	%	%
Skin prick test	≥ 95	30–60	≤ 50	≥ 95
Wheal diameter, mm				
0	4	50	18	15
≥3	95	72	91	81
≥6	78	94	98	59
≥8	51	100	100	40
Age of the child				
0	0	33	0	6
≥3	100	67	94	100
≥4	93	100	100	75
ImmunoCAP Fluoroenzyme immunoassay result ≥ 15 kUA/L (95%) predictive decision point	57	100	100	36
Food challenge*	~100	~100	~100	~100

*False-negative and false-positive results have rarely been reported with double-blind, placebo-controlled food challenges. The majority of false-negative results may occur because of ingestion of inadequate doses of food required to provoke an allergic reaction. False-positive results may be recorded if the challenge is terminated after only subjective symptoms (e.g., oral pruritus, and itchiness) have been reported.

THERAPY

Acute management. It is unlikely to be able to avoid contact with peanuts and it is possible to be accidentally be exposed to peanuts at any time. Family, personal at the school should be inform about the peanut allergy and instructed to act in emergency (to recognized the signs of the peanut allergy, to administrated adrenaline/epinephrine and to call emergency). Bracelet or equivalent that tells other people about allergy should be wear. Patients with peanut allergy must carry always an auto-injector with adrenaline/epinephrine.

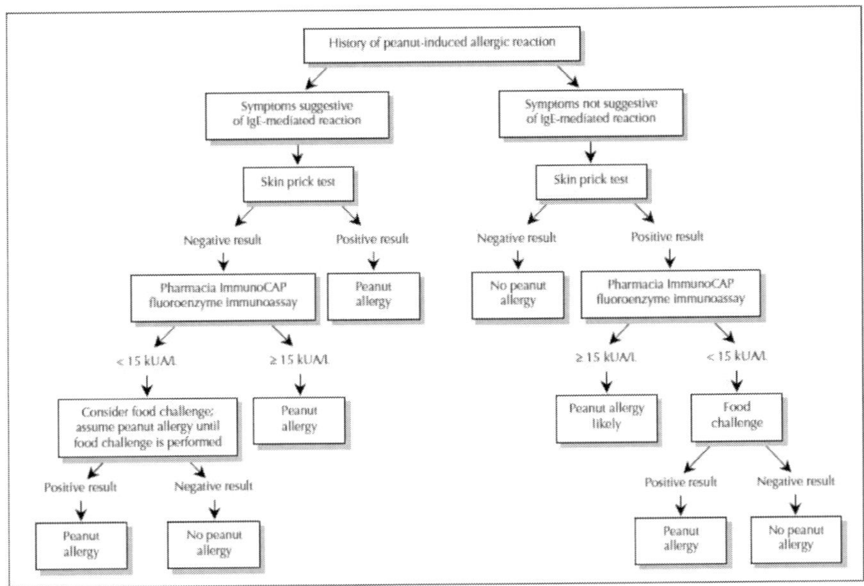

Figure 3. Algorithm for the diagnostic of peanut allergy [2].

Mild reactions (skin symptoms) can be treated with an H1 non-sedating antihistamine (e.g., loratadine, desloratadine, cetirizine, levocetirizine, mizolastine, rupatadine, ebastine, etc.) in usual dosage. Those tablets which are dispensed orally (like desloratadine) may act in 5 minutes; the others usually need 15-30 minutes to be active.

More severe reactions (respiratory, cardiovascular) are treated as emergency, as soon as possible with adrenaline/epinephrine (0.3 mg for adults, 0.15 mg for children) given intramuscularly (in the superior region of thigh). The dose may be repeated after 20 minutes (Table 4). There are auto-injectors containing the proper dosage in devices (pens like EpiPen, AnaPen, Jext, etc.). This pens should be carry all the time by the severe allergic patients or should be kept in the places where they spend most of the time.

For wheezing, a short acting beta-2-agosnist (e.g., albuterol) should be administrated (inhaled 2 to 4 puffs).

Table 4. Acute therapy for anaphylactic shock [18]

Rapid assessment of:	Extent and severity of symptoms
	Adequacy of oxygenation, cardiac output, and tissue perfusion
	Potential confounding medication
	Suspect cause of the reaction
Initial Therapy:	Epinephrine 0.01 mg/kg/dose up to 0.3-0.5 mg sc or im up to three times every 20 minutes
	Oxygen, 40%-100% by mask
	Intravenous fluids, 30 mL/kg of crystalloid up to 2 L (or more, depending on blood pressure and response to meds)
Secondary medications:	Nebulized albuterol; may be continuous
	Antihistamines (H1 antagonist – diphenhydramine 1 mg/kg up to 75 mg, preferred second generation of H1-e.g., orally absorbed desloratadine, H2 antagonist – ranitidine)
	Corticosteroids: solumedrol 1-2 mg/kg/dose iv; prednisone 1-2 mg/kg/dose, orally
	Dopamine 2-20 µg/kg/min for hypotension refractory to epinephrine
	Norepinephrine for hypotension refractory to epinephrine
	Glucagon for hypotension refractory to epinephrine and norepinephrine, especially patients with beta-blockers

If the patients does not recover it should be admitted to intensive care unit to be treated with oxygen, i.v. solutions (glucagon, saline, glucose) to reload vascular system (up to 2-4 liters), vasopressor support, mechanical ventilation.

Long Term Management

For long term management patients should be educate to identified and avoid foods containing peanuts (label, Chinese food, sweets, candies, cereals and baked goods, such as cookies, cakes and pies, etc.). In restaurants some ingredients may contain peanuts - for example, peanut butter may be an ingredient in a sauce or marinade. Especially Asian and Mexican food and other cuisines use peanuts. Even ice cream parlors may not be safe for people with a peanut allergy, since peanuts are a common topping.

Patients with severe anaphylaxis should be educate for carrying pens with epinephrine.

In the last year, therapy to induce tolerance to peanut developed (oral immunotherapy). Also studies for therapy with anti-IgE monoclonal antibodies were performed.

Oral Immunotherapy

Oral Immunotherapy is a specific therapy for allergic patients which induce tolerance to the allergen causing the diseases. Tiny amounts of the allergen are given to the patients orally which and the quantity is gradually increased over time. The aim is to build up tolerance to the allergen. This treatment has been used with success to treat cow milk allergy. At present it is not widely used to treat food allergy such as nut allergy because of the risk of anaphylaxis. Immunotherapy is given in specialized allergy centers. However, studies looking at this are underway. Promising results from different studies are published in the last 3 years [22, 23, 24].

Monoclonal Antibodies Anti-IgE

Humanized recombinant anti-IgE antibodies were used in peanut allergic patients. During this biological therapy, the patients had an increased, tolerated quantity of peanuts [25]. TNX-901 and omalizumab were used [26].

Chinese Herbal Therapy

Food Allergy Herbal Formula-2 (FAHF-2) is a 9-herb formula based on traditional Chinese medicine that blocks peanut-induced anaphylaxis in a murine model [25]. In phase I studies FAHF-2 was found to be safe and well tolerated. The conclusion of the authors was that FAHF-2 is a safe herbal medication for subjects with food allergy, but however, efficacy for improving tolerance to food allergens is not demonstrated at the dose and duration used [27].

Can Nut Allergy Be Prevented?

In the past, the Department of Health advised that atopic pregnant and breast-feeding mothers and their infants should avoid peanuts. However, in 2009, the Department of Health changed their advice.

The new published data have shown that there is no clear evidence that eating or not eating peanuts (or foods containing peanuts) during pregnancy, whilst breast-feeding or during early infant life, influences the chances of a child developing a peanut allergy.

Pregnancy/Breast-Feeding

If mothers would like to eat peanuts or foods containing peanuts during pregnancy or whilst breast-feeding, then they can choose to do so as part of a healthy balanced diet, irrespective of whether they have a family history of allergies.

When Introducing Peanut into the Child's Diet

If mothers choose to start giving their baby solid foods before 6 months (after talking to a health visitor or GP), they should not introduce peanuts or other allergens such as nuts, seeds, milk, eggs, wheat, fish or shellfish before this time. Furthermore, when these foods are introduced, they should be introduced one at a time so that they can spot any allergic reaction.

Recently, a British study (LEAP - Learning Early About Peanut Allergy) on a of 640 children, aged four months to 11 months, published the findings regarding the early introduction of peanuts [28]. The children were considered at high risk of becoming allergic to peanuts either because of a pre-existing egg allergy or eczema, which can be linked to peanut allergy. They were randomized into two groups - some were fed foods containing pureed peanuts and others were told to avoid peanuts until they turned five. They found that by age five, fewer than one percent of the children who ate food containing peanuts three or more times each week developed a peanut allergy, compared to 17.3 percent in the group that avoided peanuts entirely (Figure 4). The final results did not include 13 out of 319 randomized children who were excused after showing signs of peanut allergy early in the study. The children involved in the research were also not fed whole peanuts, which can be a choking hazard. This is an important clinical development and contravenes previous guidelines because introduce a new concept regarding early introduction of allergen in life in order to develop tolerance (instead hypersensitivity!).

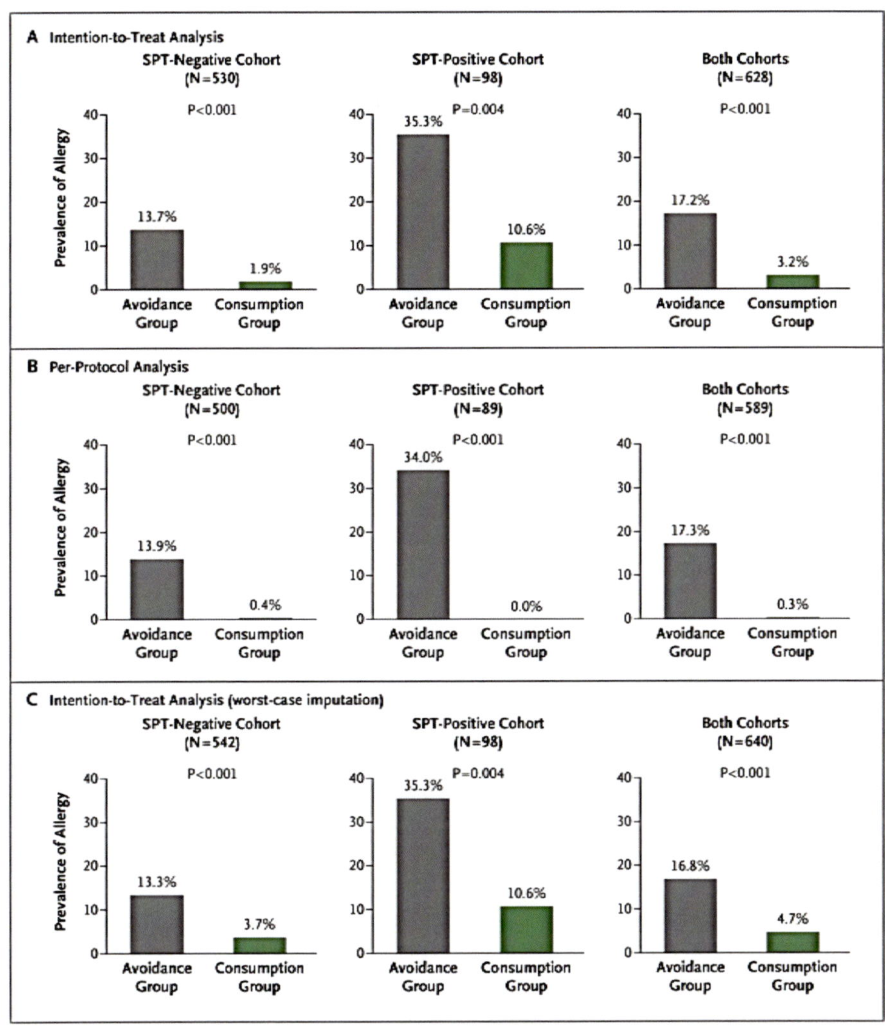

Figure 4. Early consumption of peanut increased the tolerance to peanuts [28].

Where a child has already been diagnosed with another kind of allergy (e.g., eczema or an allergy to foods other than peanut), or if there is a history of allergy in the child's family. Mothers are encouraged to talk to their GP, health visitor or medical allergy specialist before giving peanut to the child for the first time, because they are at higher risk of developing peanut allergy.

PREVENTION

For an allergic patients it is very important to avoid the allergen, to avoid peanuts and peanuts-derived products. In recent years, awareness about peanut allergy in children has risen, as has the number of peanut allergy cases reported. Many schools have declared that they are "nut-free," meaning that the onetime staple of kids' lunchboxes — a peanut butter and jelly sandwich — is nowhere to be found on school grounds these days. That's because peanuts can cause a life-threatening reaction in some people.

Foods must be labeled for traces of peanuts (according the the safety laws for labeling).

Patients with severe reaction should carry an auto-injector with adrenaline/epinephrine to be administrated in case of an unexpected reaction.

REFERENCES

[1]   Taylor, S. L. & Hefle, S. L. (2002). Foods as allergens. In Brostoff, J., Challacombe S. *Food Allergy and Intolerance*, 2nd Ed. Sauders, 403-412.

[2]   Al-Muhsen, S., Clarke A. E. & Kagan, R. S. (2003). Peanut allergy: an overview. *CMAJ*, *168*, 1279-1285.

[3]   Dyer, A. A., Rivkina, V., Perumal. D., Smeltzer. B. M., Smith. B. M. & Gupta R. S. (2015). Epidemiology of childhood peanut allergy. *Allergy Asthma Proc*, *36*, 58-64.

[4]   Skripak, J. M. & Wood, R. A. (2008). Peanut allergy and tree allergy in childhood. *Pediatr Allergy Immunol*, *19*, 368-373.

[5]   Pumphrey, R. S. H. (2000). Lessons from management of anaphylaxis from a study of fatal reactions. *Clin. Exp. Allergy.*, *30*, 1144-1150.

[6]   Yunginger, J. W., Sweeney, K. G., Stunrner, W. Q., Giannandrea, L. A., Teigland, J. D., Bray, M. B., Benson, P. A., York, J. A., Biedrzycki, L.,

Squillance, D. L., et al. (1988). Fatal food-induced Anaphylaxis. *JAMA*, *260*, 1450-1452.

[7]   Bock, S. A., Mũnoz-Furlong, A. & Sampson, H. A. (2001). Fatalities due to anaphylactic reactions to foods. *J Allergy Clin Immunol, 107*, 191-193.

[8]   Lack, G., Fox, D., Northstone, K. & Golding, J. (2003). Factors Associated with the development of peanut allergy in Childhood. *New Eng J Med, 348*, 977-985.

[9]   European Commission. Scientific Report on Consumer Safety. *Opinion on Peanut Oil (sensitization only).*, 2014.

[10]   Sporik, R., Hill, D. J. & Hosking, C. S. (2000). Specificity of allergen skin testing in predicting positive open food challenges to milk, egg and peanut in children. *Clin Exp Allergy, 30*, 1540-1546.

[11]   Sicherer, S. H., Mũnoz-Furlong, A., Godbold, J. H. & Sampson, H. A. (2010). US prevalence of self-reported peanut, tree nut and sesame allergy: 11-year follow-up. *J Allergy Clin Immunol., 125*, 1322-1326.

[12]   Sicherer S. H., Mũnoz-Furlong A. & Sampson, H. A. (2003). Prevalence of peanut allergy and tree nut allergy in the United States determined by means of a random digital dial telephone survey: a 5-year follow-up study. *J Allergy Clin Immunol., 112*, 1203-1207.

[13]   Wong, G. W. K. (2015). Epidemiology: International point of view, from childhood to adults, food allergens. In Ebisawa M., Ballmer-Weber B. K., Vieths S. and Wood R. A., eds. in Food Allergy: Molecular basis and clinical practice. Karger, Basel, 30-37.

[14]   Du Toit, G., Katz, Y., Sasieni, P., Mesher, D., Maleki, S. J., Fisher, H. R., Fox, A. T., Amir, T., Zadik-Mnuhin, G., Cohen, A., Livne, I. & Lack, G. (2008). Early consumption of peanuts in infancy is associated with a low prevalence of peanut allergy. *J Allergy Clin Immunol., 122*, 984-991.

[15]   Hourihane, J. O., Roberts, S. A. & Warner, J. O. (1998). Resolution of peanut allergy: case –control study. *BMJ., 316*, 1271-1275.

[16]   Sorensen, H. T., Nielsen, B. & Ostergaard, N. J. (1989). Anaphylactic shock occurring outside hospitals. *Allergy, 44*, 288-290.

[17]   Yocum, M. W. & Khan, D. A. (1994). Assessment of patients who have experienced anaphylaxis: a 3 - years survey. *Mayo Clinic Proc., 69*, 16-23.

[18] Burks, A. W. & Sampson, H. A. (2003). Anaphylaxis and food allergy. In Metcalfe, D. D., Sampson, H. A., Simon, R. A., eds. Food allergy: Adverse reactions to foods and food additives, 3rd ed. Blackwell Publishing Maldem, 192-205.

[19] Kagy, L., Blaiss, M. & Anaphylaxis, S. (2000). In Libermann P, Anderson, J. A., Allergic Diseases. Diagnostic and treatment, 2nd ed. Humana Press Totowa, New Jersey, 53-71.

[20] Anderson, J. A. (2000). Food allergy and Intolerance. In Libermann P, Anderson J. A. Allergic Diseases. Diagnostic and treatment, 2nd ed. Humana Press Totowa, New Jersey, 283-302.

[21] Metcalfe, D. D. (2003). Food allergy in adults. In Metcalfe D. D., Sampson H. A., Simon R. A., eds. Food allergy: Adverse reactions to foods and food aditives, 3rd ed. Blackwell Publishing Maldem, 136-143.

[22] Michaud, E., Evrard, B., Pereira B., Rochette, E., Bernard, L., Rouzaire, P-O., Gourdon-Dubois, N., Merlin, E. & Fauquert, J. L. (2015). Peanut oral immunotherapy in adolescents: study protocol for a randomized controlled trial. *Trials, 16,* 197-202.

[23] Narisety, S. D., Frischmeyer-Guerrerio, P. A., Keet, C. A., Gorelik, M., Schroeder, J., Hamilton, R. G. & Wood, R. A. (2015). A randomized, double-blind, placebo-controlled pilot study of sublingual versus oral immunotherapy for the treatment of peanut allergy. *J Allergy Clin Immunol., 135,* 1275-1282.

[24] Umetsu, D. T., Rachid, R. & Schneider, L. C. (2015). Oral immunotherapy and anti-IgE antibody treatment for food allergy. *World Allergy Organ J., 8*(1), 20-25.

[25] Leung, D. Y., Sampson, H. A., Yunginger, J. W., Burks, A. W., Schneider, L. C., Wortel, C. H., Davis, F. M., Hyun, J. D., Shanahan, W. R. for the TNX-901 Peanut Allergy Study Group (2003). Effect of anti-IgE therapy (TNX-901) in patients with peanut allergy. *N Engl J Med, 348,* 986-993.

[26] Srivastava, K. D., Bardina, L., Sampson, H. A. & Li, X. M. (2012). Efficacy immunological actions of FAFH-2 in a murine model of multiple food allergies. *Ann Allergy Asthma Immunol., 108*(5), 351-358. e1.

[27] Wang, J., Jones, S. M., Pongracic, J. A., Song, Y., Yang, N., Sicherer, S. H., Makhija, M. M., Robinson, R. G., Moshier, E., Godbold, J., Sampson, H. A. & Li, X. M. (2015). Safety, clinical, and immunological efficacy of a Chinese herbal medicine (Food allergy herbal formula-2) for food allergy. *J Allergy Clin Immunol.* pii: S0091-6749(15)00634-X. doi: 10.1016/j.jaci.2015.04.029.

[28] Du Toit, G., Roberts, G. D. M., Sayre, P. H., Bahnson, H. T., Radulovic, S., Santos, A. F., Brough, H. A., Phippard, D., Basting, M., Feeney, M., Turcanu, V., Sever, M. L., Gomez-Lorenzo, M., Plaut, M. & Lack, G. for the LEAP Study Team., (2015). Randomized trial of peanut consumption in infants at risk for peanut allergy. *N Engl J Med, 372,* 803-813.

Chapter 2

PEANUT ALLERGENS

Maria Pele, PhD* and Carmen Cimpeanu, PhD
University of Agronomic Sciences and
Veterinary Medicine - Bucharest, Romania

ABSTRACT

Food allergies have a considerable impact on modern society. Some of the most severe allergic reactions occur when peanuts and peanut derivatives are consumed. The mainly causative agents of peanut allergy are proteins. Total protein content of peanut is represented up to 32 different proteins of which about 18 (28 considering isoforms, variants and peanut lectin), nearly 7-10%, have been identified as capable of binding specific IgE, so to be allergenic. From the description of the first peanut allergen called Ara h1 in 1991 so far have been described about 28 proteins with allergenic action. So, allergenic proteins in peanut, named Ara h1 – Ara h17 and agglutinin have been identified, some largely characterized and with the exception of Ara h 16 and Ara h 17, were accepted by Allergen Nomenclature Subcommittee of the International Union of Immunological Societies (IUIS). The last two identified allergens nsLTPs are provisionally accepted and will be voted by IUIS meeting at EAACI in 2015. For some of these allergens structural features, biochemical and physicochemical properties and their biosynthesis genes encoding were established.

---

* Corresponding author: Maria Pele. Email: mpele50@yahoo.com.

Keywords: peanut, allergens

INTRODUCTION

Peanut and nut allergens represent nowadays a challenge for health and food manufacturers both. The threat of an adverse reaction can be present for sensitive people everywhere in food. Food allergy has been long recognised as a clinical phenomenon but only in the last decades a wide research was developed to identify, detect and comprehensive characterize the agents, (proteins) which provoke allergy reactions.

Peanuts are one of the 8 most common allergenic foods and a large proportion of peanut-allergic individuals have severe reactions, some to minimal exposure. The mainly causative agents of peanut allergy are proteins. Out of the total proteins in peanuts, some specific protein constituents in the peanuts are the cause of the allergic reactions in sensitized individuals who ingest peanuts. Total protein content of peanut is represented up to 32 different proteins of which nearly 7-10%, have been identified as capable of binding specific IgE, so to be allergenic. From the description of the first peanut allergen called Ara h1 in 1991 so far have been described more or less about 17 proteins with allergenic action. So were listed allergenic proteins in peanut, named Ara h1 – Ara h17 and agglutinin, have been identified, a part of them largely characterized and accepted by Allergen Nomenclature Subcommittee of the International Union of Immunological Societies (IUIS). For some of these allergens structural features, biochemical and physicochemical properties and their biosynthesis genes encoding were established.

Because, food allergy is a growing phenomenon and it is necessary a very deeply knowledge on allergens to control its. In this context, reliable detection and quantification methods for food allergens identification were used in the last 25 years. So, if in 2010 were known, clearly identified 11 allergens in peanuts, now with the development of analysis techniques, but with the necessity to know why some products, such as refined oil, produce specific consumption of peanut allergic reactions, it was given particular attention to identifying compounds of peanuts and products derived compounds that cause these reactions. Thus, up to day a total of 29 peanut allergenic compounds are known, considering all forms isoforms, variants and agglutinin.

PEANUT ALLERGENS

In peanut, nearly 7-10% of total protein content (about 25%) [1] consists of allergenic proteins (i.e., Arachine, Conarachine). Total protein content is represented by at least 32 different protein of which to date, 17 and their isoallergens have been identified as capable of binding specific IgE, so to be allergenic.

Food allergens are grouped in two classes: *class I* when the adverse reactions appear when allergen is present in the gastrointestinal tract and *class II* when allergic reactions appear to inhalant allergens. In addition, peanut allergens are *class I* allergens because they fulfil all the conditions to be included in this category, namely: they encounter the immune system through the digestive tract, they induce allergic reactions directly via the intestine, they are protein or glycoprotein, they have molecular mass between 8 to 70 kDa, they are heat stable and they are not deactivated by thermal processing, they are resistant to digestive enzymes, they are stable in acidic medium as gastric juice.

Peanut allergens are water or saline solutions soluble proteins, glycoprotein and peptides. They are seed storage and from plant defence system proteins. In peanut in compliance with the latest findings (until June 2015) have been identified the different types of peanut allergens which are listed, largely characterized and accepted by Allergen Nomenclature Sub-Committee of the International Union of Immunological Societies (IUIS) [2]. In this line the peanut allergen names are composed from the three letters of the genus scientific name (Ara), followed by the first letter of specie (h) and Arabic numerals. Because, along the time there were discovered different closely related molecular species of an allergen with similar molecular masses, similar biochemical functions and sequence identities >67%, it was introduced the designation of *isoallergens* and their identity is specified by four digits following the period after the main allergen number. The first two digits designate the isoallergen and the third and fourth distinguish different variants of an isoallergen, which are proteins with more than 90% sequence identity [3].

Thus, from the description of the first peanut allergen called Ara h1 in 1991 [4] so far have been described more or less about 30 proteins with allergenic action. These proteins have been named Ara h1 – Ara h17 and agglutinin, some of them with several isoforms. According to *Allergome* database, at present the most all-inclusive collection of allergen data, allergens could be albumins (water soluble) or globulins (soluble in dilute saline) and they are either protective, defence proteins enable to resist biotic and abiotic stress, or storage proteins. The globulins are in turn subdivided into arachin and conarachin fractions, the major storage proteins. According to the sequence relationships, structural and functional properties, more than 65% of plant proteins belong to four superfamilies: prolamin superfamily, cupin superfamily, profilin and Bet v1 families [5, 6]. Peanut allergens belongs to food allergens families as follows:

- Cupin superfamily:
- Vicillin-type, 7S globulin family: Ara h 1;
- Legumin-type, 11S globulin, Glycinin family: Ara h 3;
- Prolamin superfamily:
- Conglutin family: Ara h 2, Ara h 6; Ara h 7;
- Non-specific Lipid Transfer Protein family: Ara h 9, Ara h 16, Ara h 17;
- Profilin family: Ara h 5;
- PR-10 (Pathogenesis Related class 10 Protein), Bet v-1-related proteins: Ara h 8;
- Oleosin family: Ara h 10, Ara h 11; Ara h 14, Ara h 15;
- Defensin family: Ara h 12, Ara h 13.

For some of these allergens there were established structural features, biochemical and physicochemical properties and their biosynthesis genes encoding.

Peanut allergens could be major or minor allergens according to their capacity to bind a large amount of IgE from the majority of patients and have biologic activity. However, it was demonstrated that the most potent allergens are not necessarily those that bind the most IgE. Thus it was proposed that the major allergens should be considered on the potency of that allergen in assays of allergic effector activity and demonstration that removal of that allergen from an extract results in loss of potency [7].

The last updated information regarding peanut allergens identified and their nomenclature are presented in Table 1. The most data have been taken from the allergen, allergome, uniprot and rcsb databases [2, 8, 9, 10].

Ara h 1 is a major peanut allergen recognized by over 90% of peanut sensitive population.

Ara h 1 is a glycoprotein. It is the first peanut allergen identified [4] and the most analyzed peanut allergen. It must be stressed that this allergen is also very abundant in peanuts representing around of 12-16% of total protein. Peanut allergen Ara h 1 is included in the conarachin globulin fraction because it could be purified by using from 40% to 85% fraction of ammonium sulphate saturation [11]. The isoelectric point of Ara h 1 was first determined by Burks et al. with the value of 4.55 [4]. Subsequently, various studies have shown that this value varies within certain limits depending on the source. For example, Wu et al. showed that the value of pI is between 4.5-4.7 [12].

According to amino acid sequence, Ara h1 is a member of cupin superfamily and has high sequence similarity with other plant vicillins like Jug r 2 from walnut and Ses i 3 from sesame [13]. It is a 7S globulin or vicillin seed storage protein. Ara h1 is a highly stable symmetrical glycoprotein of three bicupins assemble highly ordered. The structure of each monomer consists of two cupin domains flanked by α-helices regions, very important for trimer formation because these are involved in the formation of oligomers assemblies. The hydrophobic residues of α-helical bundles located at the ends of each monomer contribute to the stability of the molecule. The two characteristic β-barrel domains border a central cavity held together via hydrophobic interactions. The two cupins are related to form the bicupin molecule by a pseudo two-fold axis. The three bicupins are linked by superposition of N- and C-terminal domains. In addition, Ara h 1 is a complex glycoprotein N-glycans (Figure 1). The carbohydrate content is of 2.4% [14]. It seems that the central cavities formed by the β-barrel may bind different ligands such as small molecules but not metal ions [15, 17, 18].

The major glycan species of Ara h 1 is a complex glycan containing a β-1,2 xylose attached to the proximal mannose of the glycan core and an α − 1,3 fucose residue attached to the proximal *N*-acetylglucosamine of the chitobiose core [19].

In addition it hasn't been reported that Ara h 1 to be involved in enzymatic activities although many protein having cupin folds are enzymes.

Ara h 1 has at least 23 identified allergenic epitopes of which some are immunodominant being recognized by more than 80% of patients. Some of them are located on the edges of the trimer [15] and 14 epitopes were found in the core region [20]. In fact the stable trimeric structure protects IgE epitopes from degradation under different food processing, keeping its allergenic properties even at the high temperature treatment. It is resistant to proteolytic hydrolysis too [21, 22, 23].

The molecular weight of Ara h 1 monomer has different values according to method used. Thus it was presented in literature different molecular weight such as 64 kDa [8] or 62 kDa [24].

The same situation can be found for the only one Ara h 1 isoallergen known up to date: 71.345 [25] or 68.8 [18].

Ara h 2 is a major peanut allergen being recognized by serum IgE from more than 90% of peanut allergic patients. It belongs to proteinase/alpha-amylase inhibitor family, from the prolamin superfamily, it has the recommended biochemical name Conglutin-7 and accounts for 5.9-9.3% of the total peanut protein [28]. The isoelectric point of Ara h 2 was determined in 1992 by Burks et al. with the value of 5.2 [29]. Subsequently, various studies have shown that this value varies within certain limits depending on the source or isolated isoform. So, it was showed that the value of Ara h 2 can have values of pI between 5.1-5.8 [12].

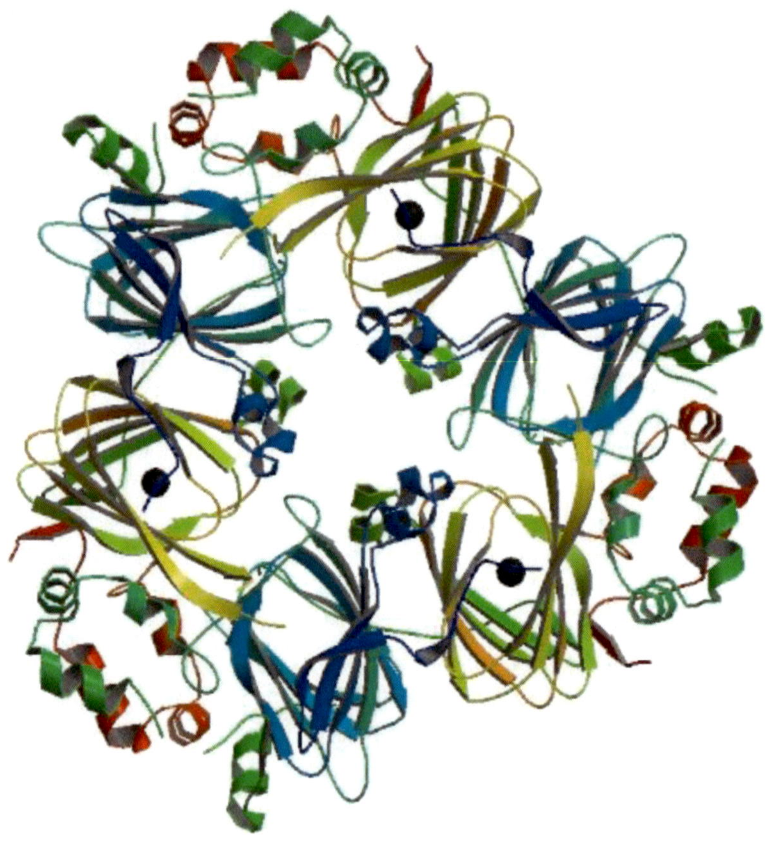

Figure 1. Crystal structure of Ara h 1 [15, 16].

Table 1. Peanut allergens identified and characterized until June 2015 [2, 8, 9, 10, 26, 27]

Allergen name	Code	Biochemical name	UniProt ID	Genbank nucleotide	MW, (SDS-PAGE), kDa	Length	pI range
Ara h 1	50	Cupin (Vicillin-type, 7S globulin)			64		4.5–4.7
Ara h 1.0101	3094		P43238	L34402	71.345	626	
Ara h 2	51	Conglutin (2S albumin)			17		5.1–5.8
Ara h 2.0101	1081		Q6PSU2-1	AY007229	20.114	172	
Ara h 2.0102	1633		Q6PSU2-2		18.700	160	
Ara h 2.0201	1082		Q6PSU2-3	AY158467	19.795	170	
Ara h 2.0202	1634		Q6PSU2-4		18.380	158	
Ara h 3	52	Cupin (Legumin-type, 11S globulin, Glycinin)			60		5.5
Ara h 3.0101	3095		O82580	*AF093541*	58.350	507	
Ara h 3.0201	10103		*Q9SQH7*	AF086821	61.011	530	
Ara h4	renamed to Ara h 3.02, number not available for future submissions						
Ara h 5	54	Profilin			15		4.6 calculated
Ara h 5.0101	3097		Q9SQI9	AF059616	14.051	131	
Ara h 6	55	Conglutin(2S albumin)			15		5-6
Ara h 6.0101	3098		Q9SQG5	AF092846	16.920	145	
Ara h 7	56	Conglutin(2S albumin)			15		5.6 calculated
Ara h 7.0101	3099		Q9SQH1	AF091737	18.418	160	
Ara h 7.0201	3928		B4XID4	EU046325	19.338	164	7.5–7.7
Ara h 7.0202	8786				17.34		

Table 1. (Continued)

Allergen name	Code	Biochemical name	UniProt ID	Genbank nucleotide	MW, (SDS-PAGE), kDa	Length	pI range
Ara h 8	1215	Pathogenesis-related protein, PR-10, Bet v 1 family member			17		≈ 5.03
Ara h 8.0101	3100		Q6VT83	AY328088	16.952	157	
Ara h 8.0201	3764		B0YIU5	EF436550	16.413	153	
Ara h 9	742	Nonspecific lipid-transfer protein type 1			9.8		9.2–9.4
Ara h 9.0101	3926		B6CEX8	EU159429	11.651	116	
Ara h 9.0201	3927		B6CG41	EU161278	9.055	92	
Ara h 10	5758	16 kDa oleosin			16		8.9–9.6
Ara h 10.0101	5759		Q647G5	AY722694	17.753	169	
Ara h 10.0102	5872		Q647G4	AY722695	15.527	150	
Ara h 11	5760	14 kDa oleosin			14		≈ 10.1
Ara h 11.0101	5761		Q45W87	DQ097716	14.308	137	
Ara h 11.0102	11752		Q45W86		14.354	137	
Ara h 12	10187	Defensin			8 kDa (reducing), 12 kDa (non-reducing), 5.184 kDa (mass)		≈ 7.7
Ara h 12.0101	10188			EY396089			
Ara h 13	10189	Defensin			8 kDa (reducing), 11 kDa (non-reducing), 5.472 kDa (mass)		≈ 7.5
Ara h 13.0101	10190			EY396019			

Allergen name	Code	Biochemical name	UniProt ID	Genbank nucleotide	MW, (SDS-PAGE), kDa	Length	pI range
Ara h 14	11753	Oleosin			17.5		-
Ara h 14.0101	11754		Q9AXI1		18.435	176	
Ara h 14.0102	11755		Q9AXI0		18.457	176	
Ara h 14.0103	11756		Q6J1J8		18.448	176	
Ara h 15	913	Oleosin			17		-
Ara h 15.0101	11757		Q647G3		16.875	166	
Ara h 16	11780	non-specific Lipid Transfer Protein 2			8.5 by SDS PAGE reducing		-
Ara h 16.0101	11781						
Ara h 17	11782	non-specific Lipid Transfer Protein 1			11 kDa by SDS-PAGE reducing		-
Ara h 17.0101	11783						
Ara h Agglutinin	1050	Galactose-binding lectin		**Gene**			-
			P02872	N/A	29.325	273	
			Q38711	lec	29.134	271	
			Q43373	lec	29.566	276	
			Q43375	lec	26.156	248	
			Q8W0P8	praiii	26.229	246	

Ara h 2 is a glycoprotein with a carbohydrate content of 20% [29] consisting of five α-helices interconnected by four disulfide bonds and arranged in a right handed super – helix. The disulfide bonds make these proteins very stable and stabilize the central core with an internal cavity where lipophilic molecules can bind [30]. The helices 2 and 3 are connected by extended 31 residue loop [17, 28, 31, 33]. This loop is sensitive to proteolysis. The main carbohydrate included in the structure of Ara h 2 is maltose. Ara h 2 has two isoallergens, each of them having two variants. These isoforms differ by their loop amino acids number and sequence [33]. The structure of Ara h 2 is similar to the proteinase/alpha-amylase inhibitors. Besides being a powerful allergen, Ara h 2 is also a weak trypsin inhibitor but its inhibiting activity increases on roasting. When the disulfide bonds are broken it decrease the protein stability, trypsin resistance as well as the allergenicity of this protein [34]. Ara h 2 contains 10 epitopes from which 3 are immunodominant [35, 36, 37]. However, it was determined that isoforms of Ara h 2 have similar epitopes but Ara h 2.0201 isoform is more allergenic than Ara h 2.0101 because the first one contain an extra immunodominat epitope, namely 3 immunodominant epitopes, while Ara h 2.0101 contains only 2 immunodominant epitopes [38]. The two immunodominant epitopes identified for both isoforms are highly immunogenic T-cell or T lymphocytes that plays a central role in cell-mediated immunity. These epitopes correspond to 19–47 (ASARQQWELQGD RRCQSQLERANLRPCEQ) respectively 73–119 (SPSQDPDRRDPYSPSPYD RRGAGSSQHQERCCNELNEFENNQRC MCE) amino acids of protein sequences.

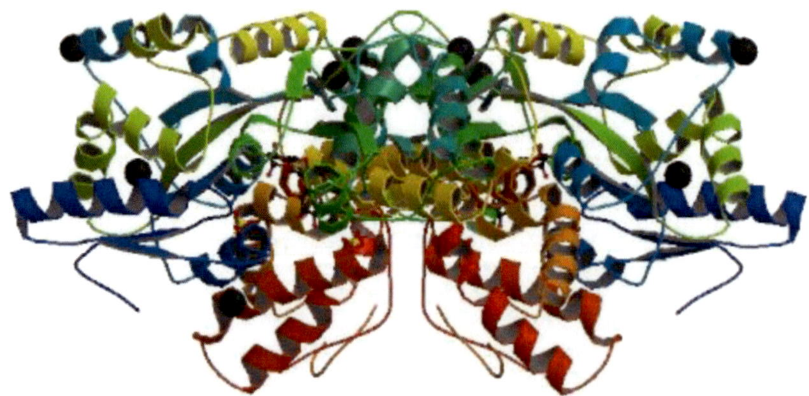

Figure 2. Crystal structure of Ara h 2 [32].

As an observation, both second variants of the two isoforms 76-87 amino acids miss (QDPDRRDPYSPS) [39]. These results are clinical relevant in order to develop a safe and effective T-cell targeted immunotherapy [40].

It must be specified that as being an albumin, it is more soluble than globulins with larger molecular mass such as Ara h 1 and Ara h 3, which it would explain why Ara h 2 and its variants account for the majority of the allergic activity in a saline extract of raw peanuts [41].

The molecular masses of Ara h 2 and its isoforms are variable according with their structure (Table 1). In addition, the variants of Ara h 2 have highly variable isoelectric points which are probably due to some posttranslational modifications.

Ara h 3 is an 11S globulin or legumin seed storage protein and belongs to cupin superfamily. It has been recognized by about 45% of peanut allergic individuals but some cultivars seems to be potentially less allergenic [42, 43]. This allergen can also function as trypsin inhibitor similar to Ara h 2 and has some role in plant defense as well [44]. Its molecular organization is typical for proteins from the glycinin family. The crystal structure of Ara h 3 is very similar to that of Ara h 1 although they shares only 21% sequence identity. However, it must be noticed that Ara h 3 shares 47.25% of sequence identity with soya bean glycinin [17, 28]. Like Ara h 1, Ara h 3 has as monomers bicupins organized in two trimers which form together a hexamer by a head to head association. Each monomer is flanked by α-helices regions, involved in the formation of oligomers assemblies, and two characteristic β-barrel domains bordering a central cavity and which held together via hydrophobic interactions. The two cupins are related to forming the bicupin molecule by a pseudo two-fold axis. The Ara h 3 protein is an 11S seed protein synthesized as a single chain with a peptide bond between the N-terminal and C-terminal domains. In the mature stage, this bond is cleaved and the hexamer is formed. The two cupin domains are acidic and basic subunits and it can be readily separated by isoelectric focusing [43, 45]. This allergen has four epitopes which are partially exposed on the monomer surface of the native allergen [47]. Of these epitopes only one is fully exposed while the other three are almost entirely covered by side chains. Because the epitopes are partially exposed on the surface of the native allergen it seems that these are only partially recognized by the IgE antibodies, which causes lower allergenicity of this allergen and it is recognized by slightly more than 35% allergic patients [28, 48, 49, 50]. In terms of molecular mass according with the method used there were determined different values, for example 57 kDa calculated using recombinant Ara h 3 or 14 kDa by immunoblots with IgE serum from peanut-hypersensitive individuals [42, 50]. The different molecular weights are due to the proteolytic cleavage. The fragments obtained have molecular mass between 14 and 45 kDa [49].

Ara h 3 has two isoallergens: Ara h 3.101 and Ara h 3.201. The isoallergen Ara h 3.201 was initially entered in the database almost in the same time with Ara h 3 as the Ara h 4, but these allergen have 91% of sequence identity. In addition both have a pI of 5.5 [42, 47, 51]. In these conditions, after the database screening by the IUIS Allergen Nomenclature Sub-Committee and based on sequences and data from the literature and in addition because the Ara h3 and Ara h4 full-length sequences shared 91.3% identity, by far exceeding the 67% identity threshold for naming isoallergen, Ara h 4.0101 was renamed Ara h 3.0201 [3].

So, Ara h 4 does not exist anymore, it was replaced by the Ara h 3.0201 isoform.

Ara h 5 is a minor allergen and only 13% - maximum 16% patients are sensitive to it. It is found in small quantities in peanut extracts. Ara h 5 belongs to profilin family and shares more of 75% and 85% similar amino acid identity with different plant from a wide range of allergens from profilin family, such as Bet v 2 (birch pollen), Gly m 3 (soya bean), Cor a 2 (hazelnut), Pru du 4 (almond) or Hev b 8 (rubber latex) [18, 52].

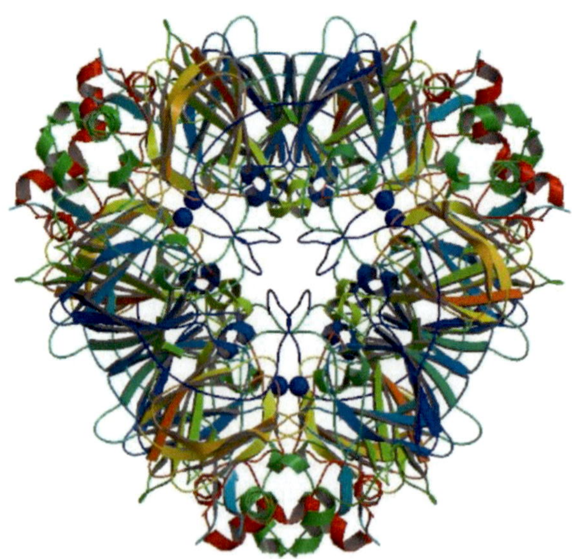

Figure 3. Crystal structure of Ara h 3 [45, 46].

Ara h 5 has a molecular weight of 15 kDa and a calculated pI of 4.6. The only isoform Ara h 5.0101 is formed by 131 amino acids and has a molecular weight of 14.051 kDa.

This allergen can act as actin-binding proteins responsible for cytoskeleton formation in plant cells and is involved in cell elongation, cell shape maintenance, polarizes growth of root hair and flowering time [17]. The structure of Ara h 5 was established and is composed of the canonical profilin α/β motif with a central anti-parallel β-sheet flanked by α-helices [53, 54, 55] (Figure 4).

Ara h 6, is a major allergen and has highly similar allergenic activity to Ara h 2 probably due to its 59% sequence identity and similar secondary and tertiary structural characteristics to Ara h 2. Thus, it was determined that 38% individuals are sensitive to this allergen [51]. Ara h 6 is composed of five α-helices and several loops fragments, flexible and disordered. Like Ara h 2, Ara h 6 has four disulfide bonds localized in the core of the molecule [17, 18, 31, 56, 57] (Figure 5). Breaking the disulfide bonds lead to a decrease of protein stability, trypsin hydrolysis resistance, as well as allergenicity [58].

Ara 6 has only one isoform with a molecular mass of 14.8 kDa and pI of 5.5 presented in allergome database. However, in different studies it has been shown that Ara h 6 has highly variable isoelectric points in the range between 5–6, fact that suggests extensive posttranslational modifications [41, 59].

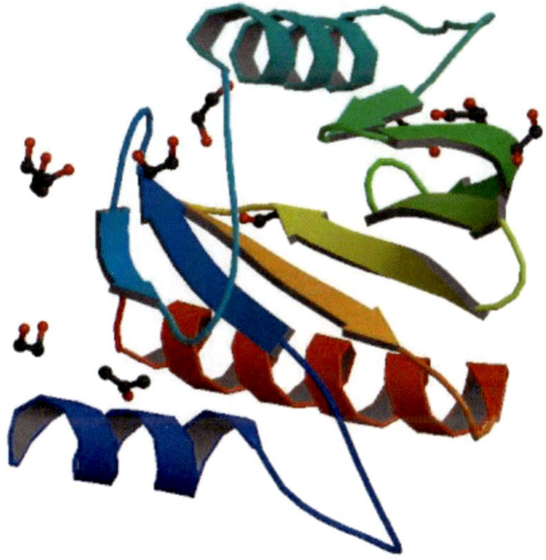

Figure 4. Crystal structure of Ara h 5 [54, 55].

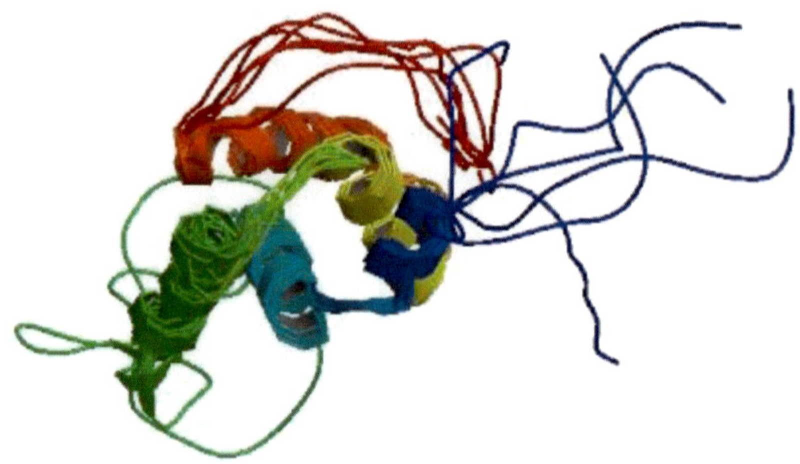

Figure 5. Crystal structure of Ara h 6 [30, 62].

Ara h 7 belongs to the conglutin family and its structure suggests that besides allergenic activity it can function as amylase or/and trypsin inhibitor. It has been recognized by 43% from 40 peanut allergic patients [51].

Currently two isoforms have been identified, one of which has two variants (Ara h 7.0101, Ara h 7.0201 Ara h 7.0202). The isoform molecular masses according to allergome database are presented in table 1 and the calculated pI of 5.6 but for isoform Ara h 7.0201 it was determined a pI of 7.5-7.7 [51, 60]. Interestingly, in accordance with the conserved cysteine pattern of conglutins, Ara h 7.0201 possesses eight cysteine residues, in contrast to the six cysteines present in the previously cloned Ara h 7.0101. Furthermore, a putative cleavage site in the Ara h 7.0202 isoform points to the characteristic biological function of conglutins as amylase/trypsin inhibitors [61].

Ara h 7.0201 show structural similarities and 42% amino acid sequence identity to Ara h 2.0201 and 43% to Ara h 6. In contrast to the allergens Ara h2 and Ara h2 which have each four disulfide bonds, Ara h 7 has only three disulfide bonds [60].

There have not been developed images of structures for allergen Ara h 7 so far.

Ara h 8 is a member of the pathogenesis – related to protein family PR – 10.

The peanut allergen Ara h 8 is very similar to birch pollen allergen Bev v 1 having 48% amino acid sequence identity and very similar structural features. So, Ara h 8 is composed of 157 amino acid residues arranged into three α-helices (two short and one long) that flank the seven-stranded anti-parallel β-sheet (Figure 6).

The central part of the molecule contains a large binding cavity composed of 30 residues, six of which are charged. In this cavity it could be linked different biological compounds such as flavonoids, lipophilic ligands or even metals [65, 66]. In addition, a Na-binding site is formed by residues connecting helix α2 and strand β2. Ara h 8 is significant thermostable that allow allergen to remain intact during food processing [63]. Although, Ara h 8 is considered to be a minor peanut allergen, due to its structure, Ara h 8 is very important for birch pollen allergic patients because of its cross reactivity with Bet v 1 [42, 67, 68]. In addition, it was observed that the severity of allergic reaction against Ara h 8 is geographically dependent and it cannot be predicted accurately [69, 70].

Ara h 8 has 2 isoforms (Ara h 8.0101, Ara h 8.0201) which have different molecular weight and pI around the estimated value of 5.03 [42]. Isoform Ara h 8.0201 is not yet in detail characterized.

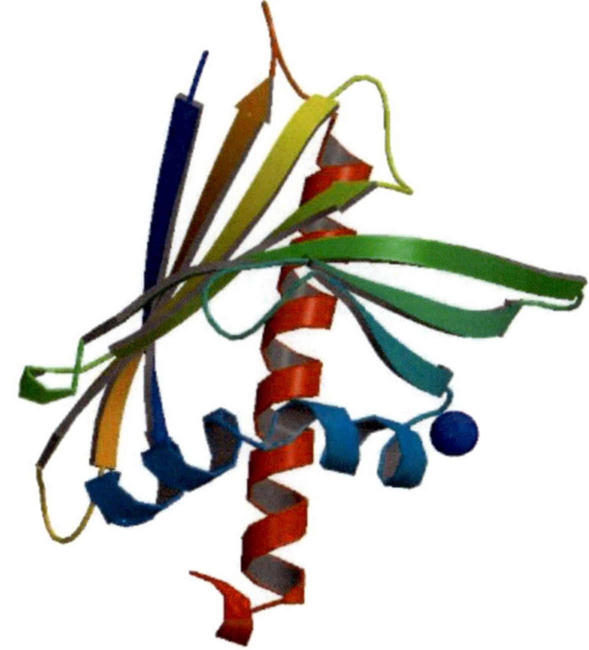

Figure 6. Crystal structure of Ara h 8 [63, 64].

The clear role of Ara h 8 in plant is not very clearly understood, but it is assumed that it is involved in defense mechanism against pathogen attacks [71].

Ara h 9 was clearly identified and partially characterized in 2009. In the early 1990s it was observed through some forensic investigations that even cooking oils could contain traces of food allergens which may be a threat to people allergic to peanuts [72, 73]. So far, it was established that nsLTPs is a very large family with representatives both in flowering and non-flowering plants except algae [74].

Proteins held responsible for these effects in oil are plants nonspecific Lipid Transfer Proteins (nsLTP). These proteins facilitate transfer of lipids between membranes *in vitro,* they have various properties in common such as: molecular masses of 9 to 10 kDa, high Isoelectric points, presence of eight cysteine residues, the ability to bind fatty acids and their derivatives and a defense role against pathogens [75, 76]. nsLTPs have ubiquitous character and they correspond to two categories of plant proteins: nsLTP1 with long chain (molecular weight 9 kDa) and nsLTP2 with shorter chain (molecular weight 7 kDa). In addition the two groups exit different disulfide bonds. Thus the disulfide bond for nsLTP1 are between Cys_1-Cys_6, Cys_2-Cys_3, Cys_4-Cys_7 and Cys_5-Cys_8 and for nsLTP2 between Cys_1-Cys_5 Cys_2-Cys_3, Cys_4-Cys_7 and Cys_6-Cys_8 [77, 78, 79]. The type I and type II nsLTPs are present across all plant species. However, in different studies the nonspecific lipid transfer proteins were classified in more types according to a system that takes into account sequence similarity and intervals of eight cysteine amino acids developed by Boutrot et al. [80]. This system categorized nsLTPs into nine types (type I–IX) based on a genome-wide analysis of rice, wheat and *Arabidopsis thaliana* (Arabidopsis). This system was subsequently applied by other researchers to different plants, sometimes with slight changes. For example, the Solanaceae nsLTPs were classified into five types (I, II, IV, IX and X) [81], to *Lotus japonicus,* into seven types (I, II, III, IV, V, VIII and IX) [82] and for *Brassica rapa* into nine types (I, II, III, IV, V, VI, VIII, IX and XI) [83]. Currently, a database contains 595 nsLTPs from 121 different species, which have been divided into five types (I-V) based on the characteristics of intervals between the eight cysteine residues, overlapping some types of Boutrot system. In addition, there is a classification based on one hand on type I and II groupings and and on the other hand on sequence similarity and glycosylphosphatidylinositol (GPI) modification site. In this classification beside the two type I and II the other nsLTPs were classified in subfamilies known as types C, D, E, F, G, H, J and K [74]. These classifications are very good resources for information concerning nsLTPs but some improvements are yet necessary [84].

The size of nsLTPs are small – approximately 90 amino acids residues, they are rich in basic amino acids which give to these allergens a pI, which usually falls between 8.5-12. Nearly all nsLTPs carry an N-terminal signal peptide directing the protein to the apoplastic space and a lot of them also carry a sequence motif for the post-translational addition of a glycosylphosphatidylinositol (GPI)-anchor [84, 85, 86, 87]. Several biological functions have been identified for plant nsLTPs such as involvement in lipid metabolism, transport of phospholipids, fatty acids, glycolipids, hydroxylated fatty acids and prostaglandin, defense activity against bacterial and fungal pathogens, resistance to abiotic stress (drought, low or high temperature, alkali, osmotic stress, hydrogen peroxide, heavy metal, light, wounding, salinization, plant hormones), involvement in cutin and wax metabolism, in seed and development and germination, in plant sexual reproduction. Some of plant nsLTPs have allergenic properties especially those from fruits (mainly from *Rosaceae*), vegetables, nuts, peanut, cereals and pollen [84, 88].

Their structure consist in four α-helices linked by four disulfide bonds and organized in a tightly packed and have a large internal cavity, tunnel-like, where it can bind a board variety of lipid types or other hydrophobic compounds. It is characterized by the eight-cysteine motif, mentioned above, forming a backbone with sequence C-Xn-C-Xn-CC-Xn-CXC-Xn-C-Xn-C, where C means cysteine and X amino acid [18, 76, 84, 89, 90].

The nsLTP from fruits have three epitopes localized on the protein surface. These allergens have an epitopic community, so, IgE-binding cross reactions frequently occur between LTP of different origin [91].

The peanut allergen Ara h 9 with its two isoforms were identified in 2008 [68, 92]. The two isoforms share 90% amino acid sequence identity and share 42%-70% amino acid sequence with LTPs from a large number of commonly foods such as hazelnut, chestnut, almond, peach, pear, plum, cherry, strawberry, lentils, lupin, sunflower, beans, pea and so on. Both of them displayed similar IgE reactivity. The Isoelectric points are 9.2-9.5 [18, 92, 93, 94, 95].

The non-specific lipid transfer protein, Ara h 9 is a major allergen at least for the sensitive people from Mediterranean area [95, 96]. The LTPs manifest high resistance to proteolytic digestion and food processing. The explanation may be that these allergens can reach the intestinal tract in an almost unmodified form [76, 97, 98]. This behaviour is determinated by the fact that LTPs are defence plant proteins against the attack of bacteria, fungi and viruses. The LTP allergy can be presented at any age [99]. Nevertheless, the last researches showed a large heterogeneity regarding the sensitivity against different allergens from peanut. In addition, it was observed that the severity of allergic reaction against Ara h 9, like for Ara h 8, is geographically dependent and it cannot predicted accurately [69, 70].

Ara h 10 belongs to Oleosin family and the biochemical name is 16 kDa Oleosin. Up to date, two isoforms of Ara h 10, namely Ara h 10. 0101 and Ara h 10.0102 have been registered in the allergome database. The molecular mass of Ara h 10 determined by SDS-Page is 16 kDa, and the two isoforms have 17.753 respectively 15.527 kDa. The purified Ara h 10 isoforms were obtained from peanut seed oil bodies where they are responsible for the formation and stability of oil bodies containing triacylglycerides. These proteins cover oil droplets (0.2-1.5 microns) in order to protect them from contacting and coalescing with other droplets. Oleosins are composed from two hydrophilic parts and one central hydrophobic core filled with lipid bodies. The hydrophobic core of about 70 residues contains a proline knot motif that is highly conserved across oleosins. The hydrophilic fragments, N- and C-terminal domains are less conserved and make the difference between oleosins. The N-terminal hydrophilic regions consists of variable length from 30 to 60 residues and the C-terminal domain consists of a variable length from about 60 to 100 amino acids residues [18, 100, 101, 102, 103]. Between the isoforms of Ara h 10 there is a sequence identity of 87%. Ara h 10 isoforms show a high sequence identity to the hazelnut oleosin Cor a 12 (56%) and the sesame oleosin Ses i 4 (42%) [60]. On the surface of hydrophilic N-terminal domain an IgE binding epitope (SDQTRTGY) was identified [104]. Besides their allergenic activity it was established that oleosins have both monoacylglycerol acyltransferase and phospholipase activities [101]. It is interesting that more than 15 years ago, Olszewski and his team were able to identify peanut allergic patients reacting to oleosins present in refined peanut oil [99]. These oleosins were divided into low and high molecular isoforms according to their basic molecular and immunological properties [106, 107, 108, 109, 110]. Very recently, using different methods of centrifugation, repeated re-solubilization, of removing the neutral lipids and purification of peanut oil body proteins, the eight peanut derived oleosins based on the sequence identity, not only on molecular masses and immunological properties, they were divided in four groups [111] called prototypes. The prototype 1 contains Ara h 10 (2 isoforms), the prototype 2 contains Ara h 11 (2 isoforms) and the prototypes 3 and 4 contain the oleosins which are included in Allergome database as Ara h 14 (3 isoforms) respectively Ara h 15 (one isoform). Their isoelectric point is alkaline and wary between 8.9 and 9.6.

The 3 D structure of these oleosins were not yet realized because appear problems due to their hydrophobicity, so their low solubility in aqueous solutions or organic solvents. Thereby to solubilize oleosins, strong detergents are needed which however, affect their structure.

Ara h 11 is oleosin with MW (SDS-PAGE) of 14 kDa. It has two isoforms (Ara h 11.0101 and Ara h 11.0102) both with the same length (137 amino acids) but with different molecular mass, namely 14.308 kDa respectively 14.354 kDa. Their isoelectric point is alkaline and it is around 10.1. The sequence identity between Ara h 11 and Ara h 10 is only 30% while Ara h 11 shows higher sequence identity to Cor a 13 (69%) and Ses i 5 (75%) [60]. Like Ara h 10, Ara h 11 besides their allergenic activity has both monoacylglycerol acyltransferase and phospholipase activities [101].

Ara h 12 belongs to defensins family, proteins rich in cysteine and small but with a large scale of activities such as fight against fungal pathogens, antibacterial, insect amylase inhibitory, protease inhibitory, cellular signalling and growth regulation [112, 113]. The peanut defensins were found in 2009 by Khodoun, et al. in a study regarding anaphylactic shock determined by peanut extract in mice. They found that a low molecular weight fraction of PE (around 5 kDa), which does not match that of any of the 8 major peanut allergens known at that time, it is particularly effective at inducing shock when injected into mice i.v. [114]. After a few years these molecules were identified and were included in Allergome database in August 2012 as peanut defensins Ara h 12 and Ara h 13. Ara h 12 has only one isoform, namely Ara h 12.0101. Thus, in lipophilic extracts obtained under alkaline conditions, Petersen et al. [115] have been found by high-resolution mass spectrometry three main peaks with monoisotopic molecular masses of 5184.1, 5200.0 and 5216.1 Da. These masses refer to the same isoform of allergen Ara h 12. The differences (differentiated by 16 mass units each) are due to the different oxidation state of the two methionine residues from the protein structure. In addition, it was clearly established that this allergen is not glycosylated. The isoelectric point is very close to neutral domain and is around 7.7.

The allergen Ara h 12 show a high sequence similarity (72%) to the pea protein Psd1 but only 43% to Ara h 13 [109, 110].

Ara h 13 belongs to pathogenesis-related protein family 12, namely the plant defensins, like Ara h 12. In lipophilic extracts obtained under alkaline conditions, Petersen et al. [115] have been found by high-resolution mass spectrometry two main peaks with monoisotopic molecular masses of 5442.4, and 5472.4 Da. The analysis of the two peaks led to the conclusion that these represent two isoforms of the allergen Ara h 13. Thus, one referred to accession number EY396019 of GenBank Nucleotide, which is registered in the Allergen Nomenclature (IUIS Allergen Nomenclature Sub-Committee since August

2012 and the other one it was found by Petersen et al. [115, 117] registered in the expressed sequence tags (EST) database with accession number EE124955. Because it was found for protein from EST database complete identity with the sequences of the peanut defensin Ara h 13 with molecular mass of 5442.4Da. Thus, it was established that Ara h 13 has two isoforms Ara h 13.0101 and Ara h.13.0102. The isoforms differ by three amino-acids. It should be noted that Ara h 13.0102 was registered in the EST in 2006 by Wan and his team, but the work by which was determined the sequence of this protein was not published [118]. However, into Allergen Nomenclature – WHO/IUIS Allergen Nomenclature – Sub-Committee, it is presented only on isoform of allergen Ara h 13, namely Ara h 13.0101. Nothing about this allergen is presented in UniProt respectively GenBank Protein databases. Like Ara h 12 nor this allergen is glycosylated. Ara h 13.0101 showed the highest sequence similarity to the Vicia faba protein ACI02060, with 70% identity [115]. The isoelectric point of the isoforms are very close to neutral domain and is around 7.5.

Plant defensins are small amphiphilic cationic proteins found in plants but also in invertebrates and vertebrates [119]. These proteins are different in their primary structure with a length of approximately 45–54 amino acids, but have a very similar characteristic three-dimensional folding pattern. The 3-dimensional structures consist of a triple stranded antiparallel β-sheet and one α-helix linked through 4 disulphide bonds between C1-C8, C2-C5, C3-C6 and C4-C7 [115, 120, 121]. The migratory behaviour in SDS-PAGe of the three peanut defensins and their allergen activity too, led to the conclusion that under natural conditions these protein form dimers. The disulphide bonds offer to peanut defensins stability against pH variations, high temperatures and proteolytic digestion [115, 116, 120].

Both peanut defensins have antifungal but not antibacterial activity. The antimicrobial activity of peanut defensins make them as interesting candidates for use in medicinal and biotechnology. So, it could be used in creams or oils for atopic dermatitis but in the meantime could be dangerous for people sensitive to peanut allergens [115]. However, plant defensins would be used for plant disease protection in transgenic crops [120, 121, 122].

Ara h 14 is an allergen that belongs to oleosin family. Its molecular mass determined by MW (SDS-PAGE) is 17.5 kDa. It has three isoforms Ara h 14.0101, Ara h 14.0102 and Ara h 14.0103. The first two isoforms (UniProt No. Q9AXI1 and UniProt No. Q9AXI0) were identified and included in the allergen nomenclature database in 2001 and the last one (UniProt No. Q6J1J8) in 2004. All data for these allergens were updated in June 2015. The isoform Ara h 14.0101 shows a sequence identity of 57% to Ara h 10.0101 and 42% to Ara h

11 [60]. The length of all these isoforms is 176 amino acids but they differ by their molecular mass 18.435 of Ara h 14.0101, 18.457 of Ara h 14.0102 and 18.448 of Ara h 14.0103. This difference is due to the presence of different amino acids in some positions. For example the isoform Ara h 14.0102 has towards Ara h 14.0101 different amino acids in positions 25, 36, 42, 142 and 163 and towards Ara h 14.0103 in positions 25, 36, 86 and 142. In the meantime the isoform Ara h 14.0103 differ towards Ara h 14.0101 only by positions 86 and 163 (Table 2) [9, 109].

Thus, the three isoforms share each other more than 97% amino acid sequence identity (Ara h 14.0102 towards Ara h 14.0101 of 97.16% sequence identity, Ara h 14.0103 towards Ara h 14.0101 of 98.86% sequence identity and Ara h 14.0103 towards Ara h 14.0102 of 97.16% sequence identity).

The allergenicity of this protein was demonstrated because this allergen has been recognized by 45.46% of from 33 peanut allergic patients [123].

Ara h 15 is also an oleosin like Ara h 14, Ara h 10 and Ara h 11. Ara h 15 has only one isoform namely Ar h 15.0101The sequence identity of this allergen to Ara h 10 and Ara h 11 is below 48% and to allergen Ara h 14 is below 30% [118]. The length of this isoform is 166 amino acids and molecular mass 16.875 kDa, while the MW determined by SDS-PAGE is 17 kDa.

It has been recognized by 45.46% of from 33 peanut allergic patients [117]. In addition it was showed in literature that Ara h 15 and Ara h 14 are potential allergens possibly associated with severe reactions [111].

Table 2. Positions of the different amino acids from the isoforms of Ara h 14 [9, 109]

	25	36	42	86	142	163
Ara h 14.0101	Proline	Isoleucine	Glutamic acid	Threonine	Valine	Glutamine
Ara h 14.0102	Glutamine	Valine	Aspartic acid	Threonine	Alanine	Glutamic acid
Ara h 14.0103	Proline	Isoleucine	Glutamic acid	Isoleucine	Valine	Glutamic acid

Oleosins can have multiple applications in the food, cosmetic or pharmaceutical industry with the condition that they be hypoallergenic. However, since the testing of the allergenicity of oleosins has just begun and these proteins are yet not in detail characterized, the lack of enough data makes it necessary future detailed studies [103].

Ara h 16 is a non-specific Lipid Transfer Protein 2. It was provisionally accepted pending on IUIS meeting at EAACI, 2015 and was just introduced in allergome database. It still has no access number neither for UniProt nor for GenBank Protein or GenBank Nucleotide database. The molecular weight of 8.5 kDa was determined by SDS PAGE reducing. The protein is 60% identical with allergen Api g 6, allergen of Apium graveolens (Celery). IgE binding to the native protein by RAST, with 16% positive out of 25 clinically proven peanut allergic subjects [125].

Ara h 17 is non-specific Lipid Transfer Protein 1. It was provisionally accepted, it will be voted on by IUIS at EAACI 2015. Protein sequence of native was de novo sequencing by LC-MSMS. Ile and Leu may be switched as masses are identical. It still has no access number neither for UniProt nor for GenBank Protein or GenBank Nucleotide database. The molecular weight of 11 kDa was determined by SDS PAGE reducing. 16% of 25 clinically defined, peanut allergic subjects had IgE binding by RAST [126].

Ara h agglutinin belongs to the large family of lectins and has as recommended name: Galactose-binding lectin, but mainly are used alternative names such as Agglutinin or PNA. Lectins are a complex group of proteins and/or glycoproteins of non-immune origin, possessing at least one non-catalytic domain which binds reversibly and specifically to monosaccharides, oligosaccharides and glycoconjugates. These proteins are found as monomers, homo- and heterodimers, as well as homo- and heterotetramer molecules. All agglutinins have a signal sequence, a peptide usually which is destined to be either secreted or part of membrane components. These signal sequences (usually 20-30) interacts with the signal recognition particle and directs the ribosome to the endoplasmic reticulum where co-translational insertion takes place, are highly hydrophobic with some positively charged amino acids. Lectins are ubiquitous proteins and there are virtually in all life forms. In plants are distributed in various tissues such as bark, bulb, fruit, latex, leaf, nodule, whole plant, phloem sap, rhizome, root, seed, stem, tissue culture, tuber, flowers and ovaries, and they have different cellular localizations and molecular properties. Plant lectins play an important role in defence mechanisms against the attack of microorganisms such as fungi, oomycetes, bacteria, and virus. Lectins are responsible for cell surface sugar recognition and have wide implications in important biological processes. Vegetable lectins display a wide repertoire of carbohydrate specificities owing perhaps to the sequence hyper variability in the loops constituting their combining site. Each lectin has a specific carbohydrate recognition highly conserved, beside this the selectivity to the other carbohydrates occurs throughout a series of weak chemical interactions such as hydrogen and/or van der Waals bonds. The diversity of biological activities conferred by lectin-carbohydrate binding, as well as the molecular structure and specificity of lectins, means that these proteins form a large and heterogeneous group. The lectins properties were studied mostly in *Arabidopsis thaliana, Phaseolus vulgaris, Amaranthus caudatus, Ricinus communis, Annona muricata, Evonymus europaea L, Nicotiana benthamiana, Erythrina speciose,* rice, wheat, pea, transgenic cotton, transgenic potato, banana and plantain, tomato, sambucus nigra, elderberry bark, rubber tree and marine alga [127, 128, 129].

The peanut agglutinin was less studied and characterized, although it has been considered as minor allergens and potential allergens for patients allergic to edible legume seeds. However, the clinical significance of the lectin-IgE interaction has to be addressed. Five iso-lectins of peanut agglutinin were identified so far. Their accession numbers to UniProtKB are: P02872, Q38711, Q43373, Q43375 and Q8W0P8. The lengths of these agglutinins vary between 246-276 with large sequences difference and the molecular masses between 26.156 and 29.566 (Table 1) with widely varied sequences. Although the overall similarity is only 42% for peanut agglutinins that correspond to the four loops that form the carbohydrate-binding site and several central residues are homologous, while others show changes to smaller side chains. The carbohydrate-binding site of peanut agglutinin may therefore have a similar peptide-backbone architecture, but form a considerably more open cleft [2, 130].

The 3D structures of peanut agglutinin complexed with different compounds such as lactose, methyl-beta-galactose, gal-beta-1,3-gal, gal-beta-1,6-galnac, gal- alpha-1,3-gal-beta-1,4-gal, gal-alpha-1,6-glc, lactose-azobenzene-4,4'- dicarboxylic acid-lactose, porphyrin, t-antigenic disaccharide, N-acetyllactosamine, different monosaccharides or polysaccharides and some peptides were realized mainly by X-Ray method. In addition, some 3D structure according to lectin-lactose complex monoclinic form, lectin-triclinic form at different pH values and ligand binding were realized. The 3-dimensional structures consist of eighteen stranded antiparallel β-sheet (five short stranded, flat six-stranded and seven curved stranded sheets) and three α-helix. The structure is similar to that in other legume lectins except in the loops. Thus, it was shown that the short five-stranded sheet plays a major role in connecting the larger flat six-stranded and curved seven-stranded sheets. Through these loops are produced two hydrophobic core, one between the two large sheets and the other one between the two ends of the seven-stranded sheet curve. It was demonstrated that 45 water molecules remain invariant when the hydration shells of the four subunits and majority of them appear to be involved in stabilising loops [131].

One of the graphic representations of peanut agglutinin forms a presented in Figure 7, in agreement with the approval of authors [131, 132].

The peanut agglutinin with the accession number UniProtKB - P02872 (LECG_ARAHY), integrated for the first time in UniProtKB/Swiss-Prot in 1986, has a homotetramer subunit structure and a three dimensional structure similarly with that presented in Figure 7. The signal peptide is 1-23 amino acids long situated at the N-terminus of protein. This protein as well, binds Mn in positions 144, 146, 155, and 160 and Ca in positions 146, 148, 150 and 155 [9, 130, 133].

The peanut agglutinin with the accession number UniProtKB - Q38711 (Q38711_ARAHY), integrated for the first time in UniProtKB/TrEMBL in 1996. The signal peptide is 1-21 amino acids long (law, 1996, uniprot.ro).

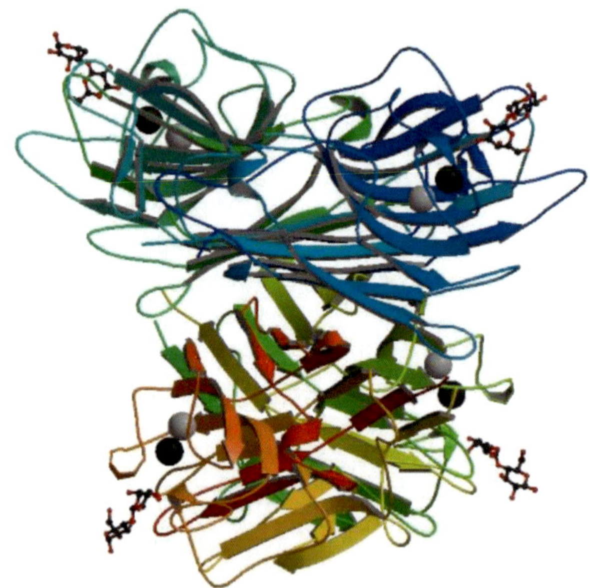

Figure 7. The structure of the complex of the tetrameric peanut lectin with lactose [131, 132].

The peanut agglutinin with the accession number UniProtKB – Q43373 (Q43373_ARAHY), integrated for the first time in UniProtKB/TrEMBL in 1996. The signal peptide is 1-21 amino acids long [9, 134].

The peanut agglutinin with the accession number UniProtKB – Q43375 (Q43375_ARAHY), integrated for the first time in UniProtKB/TrEMBL in 1996. The signal peptide is represented by one amino acid, namely serine [9, 134].

The peanut agglutinin with the accession number UniProtKB - Q8W0P8 (Q8W0P8_ARAHY), integrated for the first time in UniProtKB/TrEMBL in 2002. The signal peptide is not presented [9, 135].

The isoelectric points of the above mentioned agglutinins are not found into allergen database.

From the data presented it can be seen that the most studied form of peanut agglutinin is the one with the accession number UniProtKB - P02872 (LECG_ARAHY).

Besides the peanut agglutinin presented here, some other lectins were described for peanut but those were not entered into uniprot.org or allergome.org database and it is not also mentioned if these isoforms could have potential allergenicity [136]. In addition, into uniprot.ro database are included alongside Q43375_ARAHY and Q38711_ARAHY peanut agglutinin (which can also be found in allergome.org at allergens under the name code of Ara h Agglutinin) other four galactose-binding lectin, namely: Q43374_ARAHY, Q43376_ARAHY and Q43377_ARAHY [9].

CONCLUSION

So far the focus has been on studying the major allergens, but in recent years it has been highlighted the different properties of minor allergens given their involvement in allergic reactions. From the first peanut allergens identified in 1991, now 17 allergens in peanuts are known (a total of 27 considering isoforms and variants) plus peanut lectin which also proved to be a minor allergen. Some of peanut allergens which have been recently detected are still uncharacterised. In table it is summarised the data of peanut allergens identification and when their 3D structures were achieved.

Table 3. The peanut allergens identified and their 3D structure recorded until June 2015

	Identification References	3D Structure
Ara h 1	Burks, et al. 1991	Chruszcz et al., 2011
Ara h 2	Burks, et al. 1992	Mueller et al., 2011
Ara h 3	Kleber-Janke, T.,... 1999, Rabjohn, 1999	Jin, et al., 2009
Ara h 5	Kleber-Janke, T.,... 1999	Wang, 2013
Ara h 6	Kleber-Janke, T.,... 1999	Lehmann, 2006
Ara h 7	Kleber-Janke, T.,... 1999	-
Ara h 8	Mittag, 2004	Hurlburk, 2013
Ara h 9	Riecken, 2008; Mari, 2008	Offerman, 2015
Ara h 10	Pons et al., 2002	-
Ara h 11	Bublin, 2014	-
Ara h 12	Khodoun, 2009	Offermann, 2015
Ara h 13	Petersen, 2015	-
Ara h 14	Pons, 2005	-
Ara h 15	Vargo, 2014	-
Ara h 16	Aalberse et al., 2015*	-
Ara h 17	Aalberse, 2015	-
Ara h agglutinin	Lotan, 1975	Banerjee, 1996

In addition peanut shares many cross-reacting proteins with other members of leguminous family and that makes more difficult to detect low quantities in food. The presence of other abundant proteins can mask low abundance proteins especially in food like cookies, chocolates, sauces, etc. where the matrix it is complex. Nonetheless, individuals are sensitised to a number of allergens in a heterogeneous way, rather than stereotypically to only 1 or 2.

There is no doubt that the methods useful for allergen characterisation are complex, as allergen characterization is a difficult and troublesome task.

REFERENCES

[1] Koppelman, S. J., Vlooswijk, R. A., Knippels, L.M., Hessing, M., Knol, E.F., van Reijsen, F.C., Bruijnzeel-Koomen, C.A., (2001). Quantification of major peanut allergens Ara h 1 and Ara h 2 in the peanut varieties

Runner, Spanish, Virginia, and Valencia, bred in different parts of the world. *Allergy.* 56, 132-137.

[2]   http://www.allergome.org.

[3]   Radauer, C., Nandy, A., Ferreira, F., Goodman, Larsen, J.N., Lidholm, J., Pomes, A., Raulf-Heimsoth, M., Rozynek, P., Thomas, W.R., Breiteneder, H., (2014). Update of the WHO/IUIS Allergen Nomenclature Database based on analysis of allergen sequences. *Allergy.* 69, 413-419.

[4]   Burks, A.W., Williams, L.W., Helm, R.M., Connaughton, C., Cockrell. G., O'Brien, T., (1991). Identification of a major peanut allergen, Ara h I, in patients with atopic dermatitis and positive peanut challenges. *J Allergy Clin Immunol.* 88(2), 172-179.

[5]   Monaci, L., Visconti, A., (2012). *Allergens, in Chemical Analysis of Food: Techniques and Applications,* ed. Elsevier Inc., 693-714.

[6]   Radauer C., Bublin M., Wagner S., Mari A., Breiteneder H., (2008). Allergens are distributed into few protein families and possess a restricted number of biochemical functions. *J Allergy Clin Immunol.* 121, 847-852.

[7]   Zhuang, Y., Dreskin, S.C., (2013). Redefining the major peanut allergens. *Immunol Res.* 55(1-3), 125-134.

[8]   http://www.allergen.org.

[9]   http://www.uniprot.org.

[10]   http://www.rcsb.org/pdb/results.

[11]   Helm, R. (2001). Allergy to Plant Seed Proteins, *Journal of New Seeds.* 3(3), 37-60.

[12]   Wu, X.-Z., Huang, T., Mullett, W.M., Yeung, J.M., Pawliszyn, J., (2001). Determination of isoelectric point and investigation of immunoreaction in peanut allergenic proteins–rabbit IgG antibody system by whole-column imaged capillary isoelectric focusing. *Journal of Microcolumn Separations.* 13(8), 322-326.

[13]   Mills, E.N., Jenkins, J.A., Alcocer, M.J., Shewry, P.R., (2004). Structural, biological, and evolutionary relationships of plant food allergens sensitizing via the gastrointestinal tract. *Crit Rev Food Sci Nutr.* 44, 379-407.

[14]   Barnett, D., Howden, M.E., (1986). Partial characterization of an allergenic glycoprotein from peanut (Arachis hypogaea L.). *Biochim Biophys Acta.* 882, 97-105.

[15]   Chruszcz, M., Maleki, S.J., Majorek, K.A., Demas, M., Bublin, M., Solberg, R., Hurlburt, B.K., Ruan, S., Mattisohn, C.P., Breiteneder, H., Minor, W., (2011). Structural and Immunologic Characterization of Ara h 1, a Major Peanut Allergen. *J. Biol. Chem.* 286(45), 39318-39327.

[16] RCSB PDB ID: 3S7I - Chruszcz, M., Maleki, S.J., Majorek, K.A., Demas, M., Bublin, M., Solberg, R., Hurlburt, B.K., Ruan, S., Mattisohn, C.P., Breiteneder, H., Minor, W., (2011). Structural and Immunologic Characterization of Ara h 1, a Major Peanut Allergen. J. *Biol. Chem.* 286(45), 39318-39327. DOI: 10.1074/jbc.M111.270132; http://www.rcsb. org/pdb/images/3s7i_bio_r_500.jpg?bioNum=1.

[17] Mueller, G.A., Maleki, S.J., Pedersen, L.C., (2014). The molecular basis of peanut allergy. *Curr Allergy Asthma Rep.* 14(5), 429.

[18] Offermann, L., Perdue, M., He, J., Hurlburt, B., Maleki, S., Chruszcz, M., (2015). Structural Biology of Peanut Allergens. *Journal of Contemporary Immunology.* 2(1), 1-26.

[19] Shreffler, W.G., Castro, R.R., Kucuk, Z.Y., Charlop-Powers, Z., Grishina, G., Yoo, S., Burks, A.W., Hugh A. Sampson, H.A., (2006). The major glycoprotein allergen from Arachis hypogaea, Ara h 1, is a ligand of dendritic cell-specific ICAM-grabbing nonintegrin and acts as a Th2 adjuvant in vitro. *J Immunol.* 177, 3677-3685.

[20] Cabanos, C., Urabe, H., Tandang-Silvas, M. R., Utsumi, S., Mikami, B., Maruyama, N., (2011). Crystal structure of the major peanut allergen Ara h 1. *Molecular Immunology.* 49(1-2), 115-123.

[21] Koppelman, S.J., Bruijnzeel-Koomen, C.A., Hessing, M., de Jongh, H.H.J., (1999). Heat-induced conformational changes of Ara h 1, a major peanut allergen, do not affect its allergenic properties. *J Biol Chem,* 274(8), 4770-4777.

[22] Maleki, S. J., Kopper, R. A., Shin, D.S., Park, C-W., Compadre, C.M., Sampson, H., Burks, A.W., Bannon, G.A., (2000). Structure of the major peanut allergen Ara h 1 may protect IgE-binding epitopes from degradation. *J Immunol.* 164(11), 5844-5849.

[23] Wichers, H.J., de Beijer, T., Savelkoul, H.F.J., van Amerongen, A., (2004). The major peanut allergen Ara h 1 and its cleaved-off N-terminal peptide; possible implications for peanut allergen detection. *J Agric Food Chem.* 52(15), 4903-4907.

[24] Khan, I.J., Di, R., Patel, P., Nanda, V., (2013). Evaluating disulfide crosslinking and pH-induced aggregation of Arachis hypogea 1 as components of Peanut Allergy. *J Agric Food Chem.* 61(35), 8430-8435.

[25] http://www.uniprot.org/uniprot/P43238#family_and_domains.

[26] http://fermi.utmb.edu/SDAP/index.html.

[27] http://www.meduniwien.ac.at/allergens/allfam.

[28] Zhou, Y., Wang, J-S., Yang, X-J., Lin, D-H., Gao, Y-F., Su, Y-J., Yang, S., Zhang, Y-J., Zheng, J-J., (2013). Peanut Allergy, Allergen

Composition, and Methods of Reducing Allergenicity: A Review. *International Journal of Food Science*, Volume 2013, Article ID 9091 40, 8 pages.

[29] Burks, A.W., Williams, L.W., Connaughton. C., Cockrell, G., O'Brien, T.J., Helm, R.M., (1992). Identification and characterization of a second major peanut allergen, Ara h II, with use of the sera of patients with atopic dermatitis and positive peanut challenge. *J Allergy Clin Immunol.* 90(6 Pt 1):962-969.

[30] Dall'Antonia, F., Pavkov-Keller, T., Zangger, K., Keller, W., (2014). Structure of allergens and structure based epitope predictions. *Methods.* 66, 3-21.

[31] Lehmann, K., Schweimer, K., Reese, G., Randow, S., Suhr, M., Becker, W-M., Vieths, S., Rösch, P., (2006). Structure and stability of 2S albumin-type peanut allergens: implications for the severity of peanut allergic reactions. *Biochem J.*, 395(3), 463-472.

[32] RCSB PDB ID: 3OB4 - Mueller, G.A., Gosavi, R.A., Moon, A.F., London, R.E., Pedersen, L.C. Crystal Structure of MBP-fusion allergen. DOI: 10.2210/pdb3ob4/pdb; http://www.rcsb.org/pdb/explore/explore.do?structureId=3OB4.

[33] Mueller, G.A., Gosavi, R.A., Pomés, A., Wünschmann, S., Moon, A.F., London, R.E., Pedersen, L.C., (2011). Ara h 2: crystal structure and IgE binding distinguish two subpopulations of peanut allergic patients by epitope diversity. *Allergy*, 66(7), 878-885. doi:10.1111/j.1398-9995.2010.02532.x.

[34] Starkl, P., Felix, F., Krishnamurthy, D., Stremnitzer, C., Roth-Walter, F., Prickett, S. R., Voskamp, A. L., Willensdorfer, A., Szalai, K., Weichselbaumer, M., O'Hehir, R. E., Jensen-Jarolim, E., (2012). An unfolded variant of the major peanut allergen Ara h 2 with decreased anaphylactic potential. *Clin Exp Allergy.* 42(12), 1801-1812.

[35] Maleki, S.J., Viquez, O., Jacks, T., Dodo, H., Champagne, E.T., Chung, S-Y., Landry, S.J., (2003). The major peanut allergen, Ara h 2, functions as a trypsin inhibitor, and roasting enhances this function. *J Allergy Clin Immunol.* 112(1), 190-195.

[36] Sen, M., Kopper, R., Pons, L., Edathara, C.A., Burks, A.W., Bannon, G.A., (2002). Protein structure plays a critical role in peanut allergen stability and may determine immunodominant IgE-binding epitopes. *J Immunol.* 169(2), 882-887.

[37] Stanley, J.S., King, N., Burks, A.W., Huang, S.K., Sampson, H., Cockerell, G., Helm, R.M., West, C.M., Bannon, G.A., (1997).

Identification and mutational analysis of the immunodominant IgE binding epitopes of the major peanut allergen Ara h 2. *Arch Biochem Biophys*. 342(2), 244-253.

[38] Hales, B.J., Bosco, A., Mills, K.L., Hazell, L.A., Loh, R., Holt, P.G., Thomas, W.R., (2004). Isoforms of the Major Peanut Allergen Ara h 2: IgE Binding in Children with Peanut Allergy. *Int Arch Allergy Immunol*. 135, 101-107.

[39] http://www.uniprot.org/uniprot/Q6PSU2.

[40] Glaspole, I.N., de Leon, M.P., Rolland, J.M., O'Hehir, R.E., (2005). Characterization of the T-cell epitopes of a major peanut allergen, Ara h 2. *Allergy*. 60, 35-40.

[41] Porterfield, H.S., Murray, K.S., Schlichting, D.G., Chen, X., Hansen, K.C., Duncan, M.W., Dreskin, S.C., (2009). Effector activity of peanut allergens: a critical role for Ara h 2, Ara h 6, and their variants. *Clin Exp Allergy*. 39(7), 1099-1108.

[42] Wen, H.-W., Borejsza-Wysocki, W, DeCory, T.R., Durst, R.A., (2007). Peanut Allergy, Peanut Allergens, and Methods for the Detection of Peanut Contamination in Food Products. *Compr. rev. food sci. food saf.*. 6, 47-58.

[43] Guo, B., Liang, X., Chung, S.Y., Maleki, S.J., (2008). Proteomic screening points to the potential importance of Ara h 3 basic subunit in allergenicity of peanut. *Inflamm Allergy Drug Targets*. 7(3), 163-166.

[44] Candido E.S., Pinto, M.F., Pelegrini, P.B., Lima, T.B., Silva, O.N., Pogue, R., Grossi-de-Sa, M.F., Franco, O.L. (2011). Plant storage proteins with antimicrobial activity: novel insights into plant defense mechanisms. *FASEB J*. 25(10), 3290-3305.

[45] Jin, T., Guo, F., Chen, Y-W., Howard, A., Zhang, Y-Z., (2009). Crystal structure of Ara h 3, a major allergen in peanut. *Mol Immunol*. 46(8-9), 1796-1804.

[46] RCSB PDB ID: 3C3V - Jin, T., Guo, F., Chen, Y-W., Howard, A., Zhang, Y-Z., (2009). Crystal structure of Ara h 3, a major allergen in peanut. *Mol Immunol*. 46(8-9), 1796-1804. DOI: 10.1016/j.molimm. 2009.01.023; http://www.rcsb.org/pdb/explore/explore.do?pdbId=3C3V.

[47] Rabjohn, P., Helm, E.M.Stanley, J.S., West, C.M., Sampson, H.A., Burks, A.W., Bannon, G.A., (1999). Molecular cloning and epitope analysis of the peanut allergen Ara h 3. *J. Clin. Invest*. 103, 535-542.

[48] Rabjohn, P., C. M. West, Connaughton, C., Sampson, H.A., Helm, R.M., Burks, A.W., Bannon, G.A., (2002). Modification of peanut allergen Ara

h 3: effects on IgE binding and T cell stimulation. *Int Arch Allergy Immunol*. 128(1), 15-23.

[49] Koppelman, S.J., Knol, E.F., Vlooswijk, R.A.A., Wensing, M., Knulst, A.C., Hefle, S.L., Gruppen, H., Piersma, S., (2003). Peanut allergen Ara h 3: isolation from peanuts and biochemical characterization. *Allergy*. 58 (11), 1144-1151.

[50] Jain, A.K. (2004). Cloning and structural analysis of a cDNA encoding glycinin (Gly-1) seed storage protein of peanut. *Electron. J. Biotechnol*. 7(3), 221-231.

[51] Kleber-Janke, T., Crameri, R., Appenzeller, U., Schlaak, M., Becker, W.M., (1999). Selective cloning of peanut allergens, including profilin and 2S albumins, by phage display technology. *Int. Arch. Allergy Immunol*. 119(4), 265-274.

[52] Hauser, M., Roulias, A., Ferreira, F., Egger, M. (2010). Panallergens and their impact on the allergic patient. *Allergy Asthma Clin Immunol*, 6(1): 1.

[53] Cabanos, C., Tandang-Silvas, M. R., Odijk, V., Brostedt, P., Tanaka, A., Utsumi, S., Maruyama, N. (2010). Expression, purification, cross-reactivity and homology modeling of peanut profilin. *Protein Expr Purif*. 73(1), 36-45.

[54] Wang, Y., Fu, T. J., Howard, A., Kothary, M. H., McHugh, T. H., Zhang, Y., (2013). Crystal structure of peanut (Arachis hypogaea) allergen Ara h 5. *J Agric Food Chem*. 61(7), 1573-1578.

[55] RCSB PDB ID: 4ESP - Wang, Y., Fu, T. J., Howard, A., Kothary, M. H., McHugh, T. H., Zhang, Y., (2013). Crystal structure of peanut (Arachis hypogaea) allergen Ara h 5. *J Agric Food Chem*. 61(7), 1573-1578. DOI: 10.1021/jf303861p; http://www.rcsb.org/pdb/explore/explore.do?structureId=4ESP.

[56] Chen, X., Wang, Q., El-Mezayen, R., Zhuang, Y., Dreskin, S. C. (2013). Ara h 2 and Ara h 6 have similar allergenic activity and are substantially redundant. *Int Arch Allergy Immunol*. 160(3), 251-258.

[57] Koid, A. E., Chapman, M. D., Hamilton, R. G., Van Ree, R., Versteeg, S. A., Dreskin, S. C., Koppelman, S. J., Wuenschmann, S. (2014). Ara h 6 Complements Ara h 2 as an Important Marker for IgE Reactivity to Peanut. *J Agric Food Chem*. 6291), 206-213.

[58] Hazebrouck, S., Guillon, B., Drumare, M. F., Paty, E., Wal, J. M., Bernard, H. (2012). Trypsin resistance of the major peanut allergen Ara h 6 and allergenicity of the digestion products are abolished after selective disruption of disulfide bonds. *Mol Nutr Food Res*. 56(4), 548-557.

[59] Suhr, M., Wicklein, D., Lepp, U., Becker, W., (2004). Isolation and characterization of natural Ara h 6: evidence for a further peanut allergen with putative clinical relevance based on resistance to pepsin digestion and heat. *Mol Nutr Food Res.* 48(5), 390-399.

[60] Bublin, M., Breiteneder, H. (2014). Cross-reactivity of peanut allergens. *Curr Allergy Asthma Rep.* 14(4), 426.

[61] Schmidt, H., Krause, S., Gelhaus, C., Petersen, A., Janssen, O., Becker, W.M., (2010). Detection and structural characterization of natural Ara h 7, the third peanut allergen of the 2S albumin family. *J Proteome Res.* 9(7), 3701-3709.

[62] RCSB PDB ID: 1W2Q - Lehmann, K., Schweimer, K., Reese, G., Randow, S., Suhr, M., Becker, W-M., Vieths, S., Rösch, P., (2006). Structure and stability of 2S albumin-type peanut allergens: implications for the severity of peanut allergic reactions. *Biochem J.*, 395(3), 463-472. DOI:10.2210/pdb1w2q/pdb; http://www.rcsb.org/pdb/explore/ explore.do?structureId=1W2Q.

[63] Hurlburt, B. K., Offermann, L. R., McBride, J. K., Majorek, K. A., Maleki, S. J., Chruszcz, M., (2013). Structure and function of the peanut panallergen Ara h 8. *J Biol Chem.* 288(52), 36890-36901.

[64] RCSB PDBe ID: 4M9B - Hurlburt, B. K., Offermann, L. R., McBride, J. K., Majorek, K. A., Maleki, S. J., Chruszcz, M., (2013). Structure and function of the peanut panallergen Ara h 8. *J Biol Chem.* 288(52), 36890-36901. doi: 10.1074/jbc.M113.517797; http://www.ebi.ac. uk/pdbe/entry/pdb/4M9B.

[65] Jain, S., Kumar, D., Jain, M., Chaudhary, P., Deswal, R., Sarin, N.B., (2012). Ectopic overexpression of a salt stress-induced pathogenesis-related class 10 protein (PR10) gene from peanut (Arachis hypogaea L.) affords broad spectrum abiotic stress tolerance in transgenic tobacco. *Plant Cell Tiss Organ Cult.* 109(1), 19-31.

[66] Petersen, A., Rennert, S., Kull, S., Becker, W. M., Notbohm, H., Goldmann, T., Jappe, U. (2014). Roasting and lipid binding provide allergenic and proteolytic stability to the peanut allergen Ara h 8. *Biol Chem.* 395(2), 239-250.

[67] Mittag, D., Akkerdaas, J., Ballmer-Weber, B. K., Vogel, L., Wensing, M., Becker, W. M., Koppelman, S. J., Knulst, A. C., Helbling, A., Hefle, S. L., Van Ree, R., Vieths, S., (2004). Ara h 8, a Bet v 1-homologous allergen from peanut, is a major allergen in patients with combined birch pollen and peanut allergy. *J Allergy Clin Immunol.* 114(6), 1410-1417.

[68] Riecken, S., Lindner, B., Petersen, A., Jappe, U., Becker, W. M., (2008). Purification and characterization of natural Ara h 8, the Bet v 1 homologous allergen from peanut, provides a novel isoform. *Biol Chem.* 389(4), 415-423.

[69] Klemans, R. J., van Os-Medendorp, H., Blankestijn, M., Bruijnzeel-Koomen, C. A., Knol, E. F., Knulst, A. C., (2015). Diagnostic accuracy of specific IgE to components in diagnosing peanut allergy: a systematic review. *Clin Exp Allergy.* 45(4), 720-730.

[70] Glaumann, S., Nopp, A., Johansson, S. G., Borres, M. P., Lilja, G., Nilsson, C., (2013). Anaphylaxis to peanuts in a 16-year-old girl with birch pollen allergy and with monosensitization to Ara h 8. *J Allergy Clin Immunol Pract.* 1(6), 698-699.

[71] Fernandes, H., Michalska, K., Sikorski, M., and Jaskolski, M., (2013). Structural and functional aspects of PR-10 proteins. *FEBS J.* 280(5), 1169-1199.

[72] Hoffman D.R., Collins-Williams, C., (1994). Cold-pressed peanut oils may contain peanut allergen. *J Allergy Clin Immunol.* 93(4), 801-802.

[73] Hourihane, J.O., Bedwani, S.J. Dean, T.P., Warner, J.O., (1997). Randomised, double blind, crossover challenge study of allergenicity of peanut oils in subjects allergic to peanuts. *BMJ.* 314(7087), 1084-1088.

[74] Edstam, M.M., Viitanen, L., Salminen, T.A., Edqvist, J., (2011). Evolutionary history of the non-specific lipid transfer proteins. *Mol Plant.* 4, 947-964.

[75] Kader, J.C., (1996). Lipid-Transfer Proteins in Plants. *Annu Rev Plant Physiol Plant Mol Biol.* 47, 627-654.

[76] Salcedo, G., Sanchez-Monge, R., Barber, D., Diaz-Perales, A., (2007). Plant non-specific lipid transfer proteins: an interface between plant defence and human allergy. *Biochim Biophys Acta.* 1771(6), 781-791.

[77] Hoh, F., Pons, J.L., Gautier, M.F., de Lamotte, F., and Dumas, C., (2005). Structure of a liganded type 2 non-specific lipid-transfer protein from wheat and the molecular basis of lipid binding. *Acta Crystallogr. D Biol.* 61, 397-406.

[78] Pasquato, N., Berni, R., Folli, C., Folloni, S., Cianci, M., Pantano, S., Helliwell, J.R., Zanotti, G., (2006). Crystal structure of peach Pru p 3, the prototypic member of the family of plant non-specific lipid transfer protein pan-allergens. *J. Mol. Biol.* 356, 684-694.

[79] Wang, N-J., Lee, C-C., Cheng, C-S., Lo, W-C., Yang, Y-F., Chen, M-N., Lyu, P-C., (2012). Construction and analysis of a plant non-specific lipid transfer protein database (nsLTPDB). *BMC Genomics.* 13(Suppl. 1):S9.

[80] Boutrot, F., Chantret, N., Gautier, M.F., (2008). Genome-wide analysis of the rice and Arabidopsis non-specific lipid transfer protein (nsLtp) gene families and identification of wheat nsLtp genes by EST data mining. *BMC Genomics*. 9, 86-105.

[81] Liu, W., Huang, D., Liu, K., Hu, S., Yu, J., Gao, G., Song, S., (2010). Discovery, Identification and Comparative analysis of non-specific lipid transfer protein (nsLTP) family in Solanaceae. *Genomics, Proteomics and Bioinformatics*. 8, 229-237.

[82] Tapia, G., Morales-Quintana, L., Parra, C., Berbel, A., Alcorta, M., (2013). Study of nsLTPs in Lotus japonicus genome reveal a specific epidermal cell member (LjLTP10) regulated by drought stress in aerial organs with a putative role in cutin formation. *Plant Molecular Biology*. 82, 485-501.

[83] Li, J., Gao, G., Xu, K., Chen, B., Yan, G., Li, F., Qiao, J., Zhang, T., Wu, X., (2014). Genome-wide survey and expression analysis of the putative non-specific lipid transfer proteins in Brassica rapa. L. *PLoS One*. 9, e84556.

[84] Liu, F., Zhang, X., Lu, C., Zeng, X., Li, Y., Fu, D., Wu, G., (2015). Non-specific lipid transfer proteins in plants: presenting new advances and an integrated functional analysis. *Journal of Experimental Botany*. doi:10.1093/jxb/erv313, http://jxb.oxfordjournals.org/.

[85] DeBono, A., Yeats, T.H., Rose, J.K., Bird, D., Jetter, R., Kunst, L., Samuels, L., (2009). Arabidopsis LTPG is a glycosylphosphatidylinositol-anchored lipid transfer protein required for export of lipids to the plant surface. *Plant Cell*. 21, 1230-1238.

[86] Lee, S.B., Go, Y.S., Bae, H.J., Park, J.H., Cho, S.H., Cho, H.J., Lee, D.S., Park, O.K., Hwang, I., Suh, M.C., (2009). Disruption of glycosylphosphatidylinositol-anchored lipid transfer protein gene altered cuticular lipid composition, increased plastoglobules and enhanced susceptibility to infection by the fungal pathogen, Alternaria brassicicola. *Plant Physiol*. 150, 42-54.

[87] Ambrose, C., DeBono, A., Wasteneys, G., (2013) Cell Geometry Guides the Dynamic Targeting of Apoplastic GPI-Linked Lipid Transfer Protein to Cell Wall Elements and Cell Borders in Arabidopsis thaliana. *PLoS ONE*. 8(11): e81215.

[88] Gadermaier, G., (2014) Non-specific lipid transfer proteins – a protein family in search of an allergenic pattern. *Int Arch Allergy Immunol*. 164, 169-170.

[89] José-Estanyol, M., Gomis-Rüth, F.X., Puigdomènech, P., (2004). The eight cysteine motif, a versatile structure in plant proteins. *Plant Physiology and Biochemistry.* 42, 355-365.

[90] Sigrist, C.J.A., Cerutti, L., de Castro, E., Langendijk-Genevaux, P.S., Bulliard, V., Bairoch, A., Hulo, N., (2010). PROSITE, a protein domain database for functional characterization and annotation. *Nucleic Acids Res.* 38:D161-D166.

[91] Rouge, P., Borges, J-P., Culerrier, R., Brule, C., Didier, A. Barre, A., (2009). Les proteines de transfert des lipides: des allergenes importants des fruits. *Revue française d'allergologie.* 49, 58-61.

[92] Mari, A., Riecken, S, Quaratino, D, Zennaro, D, Reese, G, Petersen, A, Vieths, S, Becker, W., (2008). Identification of a Lipid Transfer Protein (LTP) in Peanut Extract and Cloning of Two LTP Isoallergens. *Journal of Allergy and Clinical Immunology.* 121(2), S212-S212.

[93] Breiteneder, H., Mills, C., (2005). Nonspecific lipid-transfer proteins in plant foods and pollens: an important allergen class. *Curr Opin Allergy Clin Immunol.* 5(3), 275-279.

[94] Krause, S., Reese, G., Randow, S., Zennaro, D., Quaratino, D., Palazzo, P., Ciardiello, M.A., Petersen, A., Becker, W.M., Mari, A., (2009). Lipid transfer protein (Ara h 9) as a new peanut allergen relevant for a Mediterranean allergic population. *J. Allergy Clin. Immunol.* 124,771-778.

[95] Lauer, I., Dueringer, N., Pokoj, S., Rehm, S., Zoccatelli, G., Reese, G., Moncin, M., Bahima, C., Enrique, E., Lidholm, J., Vieths, S., Scheurer, S., (2009). The non-specific lipid transfer protein, Ara h 9, is an important allergen in peanut. *Clin. Exp. Allergy.* 39(9), 1427-1437.

[96] Romano, A., Fernandez-Rivas, M. Caringi, M., Amato, S., Mistrello, G., Asero, R., (2009). Allergy to peanut lipid transfer protein (LTP): frequency and cross-reactivity between peanut and peach LTP. *Eur Ann Allergy Clin Immunol.* 41(4), 106-111.

[97] Asero, R., Mistrello, G. Roncarolo, D., de Vries, S.C., Gautier, M.F., Ciurana, C.L., Verbeek, E., Mohammadi, T., Knul-Brettlova, V., Akkerdaas, J.H., Bulder, I., Aalberse, R.C., van Ree, R., (2001). Lipid transfer protein: a pan-allergen in plant-derived foods that is highly resistant to pepsin digestion. *Int. Arch. Allergy Immunol.* 124(1-3), 67-69.

[98] Asero, R., Mistrello, G. Roncarolo, D., Amato, S, (2004). Relationship between peach lipid transfer protein specific IgE levels and hypersensitivity to non-Rosaceae vegetable foods in patients allergic to lipid transfer protein. *Ann Allergy Asthma Immunol.* 92(2), 268-72.

[99] Alessandri, C., Zennaro, D., Zaffiro, A., Mari, A, (2009). Molecular allergology approach to allergic diseases in the paediatric age. *Ital. J Pediatr.* 35(1): 29.

[100] Murphy, D.J., Keen, J.N., O'Sullivan, J.N., Au, D.M., Edwards, E.W., Jackson, P.J., Cummins, I., Gibbons, T., Shaw, C.H., Ryan, A.J., (1991). A class of amphipathic proteins associated with lipid storage bodies in plants. Possible similarities with animal serum apolipoproteins. *Biochimica et Biophysica Acta.* 1088(1), 86-94.

[101] Parthibane, V., Rajakumari, S., Venkateshwari, V., Iyappan, R., Rajasekharan, R., (2012). Oleosin is bifunctional enzyme that has both monoacylglycerol acyltransferase a phospholipase activities. *J Biol. Chem.* 287(3), 1946-1954.

[102] Fang, Y., Zhu, R-L., Mishler, B.D., (2014). Evolution of Oleosin in Land Plants. *PLoS ONE.* 9(8): e103806.

[103] Vargo, K.B., Sood, N., Moeller, T.D., Heiney, P.A., Hammer, D.A., (2014). Spherical Micelles Assembled from Variants of Recombinant Oleosin. *Langmuir.* 30 (38), 11292-11300.

[104] Kobayashi, S., Katsuyama, S., Wagatsuma, T., Okada, S., Tanabe, S., (2012). Identification of a new IgEbinding epitope of peanut oleosin that cross-reacts with buckwheat. *Biosci Biotechnol Biochem.* 76(6), 1182-1188.

[105] Olszewski, A., Pons, L., Moutété, F., Aimone-Gastin, I., Kanny, G., Moneret-Vautrin, D.A. Guéant, J.L., (1998). Isolation and characterization of proteic allergens in refined peanut oil. *Clin Exp Allergy.* 28(7), 850-859.

[106] Tzen, J.T.C., Lai, Y.-K., Chan, K.-L., Huang, A.H.C., (1990). Oleosin Isoforms of High and Low Molecular Weights Are Present in the Oil Bodies of Diverse Seed Species. *Plant Physiology.* 94(3), 1282-1289.

[107] Tzen, J., Cao, Y., Laurent, P., Ratnayake, C., Huang, A., (1993). Lipids, Proteins, and Structure of Seed Oil Bodies from Diverse Species. *Plant Physiology.* 101(1), 267-276.

[108] Pons, L., Chery C., Romano, A., Namour, F., Artesani, M.C., Guéant, J.-L., (2002). The 18 kDa peanut oleosin is a candidate allergen for IgE-mediated reactions to peanuts. *Allergy.* 57 Suppl. 72: 88-93.

[109] Pons, L., Chery, C., Mrabet, N., Schohn, H., Lapicque, F., Gueant, J.L., (2005). Purification and cloning of two high molecular mass isoforms of peanut seed oleosin encoded by cDNAs of equal sizes. *Plant Physiol Biochem.* 43(7), 659-668.

[110] Jolivet, P., Acevedo, F., Boulard, C., d'Andréa, S., Faure, J.-D., Kohli, A., Nesi, N., Valot, B., Chardot, T., (2013). Crop seed oil bodies: From challenges in protein identification to an emerging picture of the oil body proteome. *Proteomics*. 13, 1836-1849.

[111] Schwager, C., Kull1, S., Krause1, S., Schocker, F., Petersen, A., Becker, W-M., Jappe, U., (2015). Development of a Novel Strategy to Isolate Lipophilic Allergens (Oleosins) from Peanuts. *PLoS ONE*. 10(4):e0123419.

[112] Okuda, S., Tsutsui, H., Shiina, K., Sprunck, S., Takeuchi, H., Yui, R., Kasahara, R. D., Hamamura, Y., Mizukami, A., Susaki, D., Kawano, N., Sakakibara, T., Namiki, S., Itoh, K., Otsuka, K., Matsuzaki, M., Nozaki, H., Kuroiwa, T., Nakano, A., Kanaoka, M. M., Dresselhaus, T., Sasaki, N., Higashiyama, T., (2009). Defensin-like polypeptide LUREs are pollen tube attractants secreted from synergid cells. *Nature*. 458(7236), 357-361.

[113] Stotz, H. U., Spence, B., Wang, Y., (2009). A defensin from tomato with dual function in defense and development. *Plant Mol Biol*, 71(1-2), 131-143.

[114] Khodoun, M., Strait, R., Orekov, T., Hogan, S., Karasuyama, H., De'Broski R.H., Köhl, J., Finkelman, F.D., (2009). Peanuts can contribute to anaphylactic shock by activating complement. *J Allergy Clin Immunol*. 123(2), 342-351.

[115] Petersen, A., Kull, S., Rennert, S., Becker, W-M., Susanne Krause, S., Ernst, M., Gutsmann, T., Bauer, J., Lindner, B., Jappe, U., (2015). Peanut defensins: Novel allergens isolated from lipophilic peanut extract. *J Allergy Clin Immunol*. 9 June − in press, DOI: http://dx.doi.org/10.1016/j.jaci.2015.04.010.

[116] de Medeiros, L.N., Angeli, R., Sarzedas, C.G., Barreto-Bergter, E., Valente, A.P., Kurtenbach, E., Almeida, F.C.L., (2010). Backbone dynamics of the antifungal Psd1 pea defensin and its correlation with membrane interaction by NMR spectroscopy. *Biochimica et Biophysica Acta (BBA)*. 1798(2), 105-113.

[117] http://www.allergen.org/search.php?Species=Arachis%20hypogaea.

[118] Wan,S.B., Bi,Y.P., Shan,L., Su,L., Quan,X.Q., Zhang,H.T., Zhang,X.Q., Lu,C.X., Zhai,H.D., Xia,M., (2006). Expressed sequence tags from an Arachis hypogaea seeds full length cDNA library. *Unpublished* http://www.metalife.com/Genbank/116489146.

[119] Thomma, B.P., Cammue, B.P., Thevissen, K., (2002). Plant defensins. *Planta*. 216, 193-202.

[120] Lay, F.T., Mills, G.D., Poon, I.K., Cowieson, N.P., Kirby, N., Baxter, A.A., van der Weerden, N.L., Dogovski, C., Perugini, M.A., Anderson, M.A., Marc Kvansakul, M., Hulett, M.D., (2012). Dimerization of plant defensin NaD1 enhances its antifungal activity. *J Biol. Chem.* 287(24), 19961-19972.

[121] Lacerda, A.F., Vasconcelos, É.A.R., Pelegrini, P.B., Grossi de Sa, M.F., (2014) Antifungal defensins and their role in plant defense. *Front. Microbiol.* 5:116.

[122] Jung, Y-J., Kwon-Kyoo Kang, K-K., (2014). Application of Antimicrobial Peptides for Disease Control in Plants. *Plant Breed. Biotech.* 2(1):1~13.

[123] http://www.allergen.org/viewallergen.php?aid=827.

[124] http://www.allergen.org/viewallergen.php?aid=828.

[125] http://www.allergen.org/viewallergen.php?aid=830.

[126] http://www.allergen.org/viewallergen.php?aid=831.

[127] Weis, W.I.; Drickamer, K., (1996). Structural basis of lectin-carbohydrate recognition. *Ann. Rev. Biochem.* 1996, 65, 441-473.

[128] Sharma, V.; Surolia, A., (1997). Analyses of carbohydrate recognition by legume lectins: Size of the combining site loops and their primary specificity. *J. Mol. Biol.* 267, 433-445.

[129] de Oliveira Dias, R., dos Santos Machado, L., Ludovico Migliolo, L., Franco, O.F., (2015). Insights into Animal and Plant Lectins with Antimicrobial Activities. *Molecules.* 20, 519-541.

[130] Young, N.M., Johnston, R.A.Z., Watson, D.C., (1991). The amino acid sequence of peanut agglutinin. *Eur. J. Biochem.* 196, 631-637.

[131] Banerjee, R., Das, K., Ravishankar, R., Suguna, K., Surolia, A., Vijayan, M., (1996). Conformation, protein-carbohydrate interactions and a novel subunit association in the refined structure of peanut lectin-lactose complex. *J. Mol. Biol.* 259, 281-296.

[132] RCSB PDB ID: 2PEL - Banerjee, R., Das, K., Ravishankar, R., Suguna, K., Surolia, A., Vijayan, M., (1996). Conformation, protein-carbohydrate interactions and a novel subunit association in the refined structure of peanut lectin-lactose complex. J.Mol.Biol. 259, 281-296. DOI: 10.1006/jmbi.1996.0319; http://www.rcsb.org/pdb/explore/ explore.do? structureId=2PEL.

[133] Ravishankar, R., Suguna, K., Surolia, A., Vijayan, M., (1999). Structures of the complexes of peanut lectin with methyl- -galactose and N-acetyllactosamine and a comparative study of carbohydrate binding in

Gal/GalNAc-specific legume lectins. *Acta Crystallographica Section D.* 55(8), 1375-1382.

[134] Law, I.J., (1996). Cloning and expression of cDNA for galactose-binding lectin from peanut nodules. *Plant Science.* 115(1), 71-79.

[135] Shanker, S., Das, R.H., (2001). Identification of a cDNA clone encoding for a galactose-binding lectin from peanut (Arachis hypogaea) seedling roots. *Biochimica et Biophysica Acta (BBA).* 1568(1), 105-110.

[136] Agrawal, P., Kumar, S., Das, H.R., (2010). Mass spectrometric characterization of isoform variants of peanut (Arachis hypogaea) stem lectin (SL-I). *Journal of Proteomics.* 73(6), 1573-1586.

ISBN: 978-1-63484-742-1
© 2016 Nova Science Publishers, Inc.

Chapter 3

PEANUT ALLERGENS CROSS REACTIVITY AND STABILITY

***Carmen Cimpeanu, PhD and Maria Pele, PhD**[*]*

University of Agronomic Sciences and Veterinary Medicine Bucharest,
Bucharest, Romania

ABSTRACT

The peanut allergens have different cross-reactions among themselves but, also with other allergens such as, for example, those of soya bean, peas, lima beans, green beans, chickpeas, lentils or other beans, pollen, nuts and even with latex. Being proteins, peanut allergens can suffer some modifications during food processing and digestion (acylation, polymerization, nitration, Maillard reaction, etc.), interactions within complex food matrices (both natural and fabricated structures). These modifications can reduce or increase their allergenic properties and are influenced by the food matrix.

Keywords: peanuts, cross-reactivity, thermal and digestion resistance, matrix effect

---

[*] Corresponding author: Maria Pele. Email: mpele50@yahoo.com.

INTRODUCTION

The allergy to peanuts (*Arachis hypogea*) is one of the most common in industrialized societies. The most fatal food allergy reactions are caused by unintentional ingestion of peanuts or tree nuts. Despite increased awareness and attention of the sensitive people, accidental exposures continue to occur at home, in restaurants or other food establishments, bakeries, ice cream shops, friend parties or other various occasions. In fact it is very difficult to track along the supply food chain avoidance of contamination by the various allergens. For example, peanut allergens could very easy cross contaminate ice creams, sauces, breakfast cereals, Asian and vegetarian foods, cookies or chocolates during production.

On the other hand, the peanut allergens are extremely resistant to various manufacturing processes so that, their ability to trigger allergic reactions is significant even after heat, enzymatic, ultrasonic or high pressure treatment.

Because there is no cure for peanut allergy, allergic people must strictly avoid peanut or possible contaminated foods.

CROSS REACTIVITY

One problem that arises for people sensitive to peanuts is that they can have allergic reactions over other foods too due to cross-reactivity phenomenon. It is very important that in assessing allergy patients must also consider the cases where co-sensitization phenomenon occurs, where the allergic reactions are not due to cross–reactivity but, to multiple sensitizations, so patient with allergies to many different molecules from different sources and their immunological reactivity can be evaluated using different criteria. In fact it is hard to predict whether a peanut allergic patient will have cross reactive reactions to similar proteins from other foods. Therefore each patient should be assessed specifically but taking into account and the results of research on aspects of cross reactivity of molecules.

The cross-reactivity is an immunological phenomenon whose clinical manifestation (when this occurs) is the association of 2 or more allergies and is due to the similarity of structural properties of the proteins involved, mainly by primary and tertiary structural similarities. Thus, plant proteins which have similar functions can have structural similarities and may have similar allergens structures. Different proteins have one or more regions recognized and bound by an antibody. These regions are named epitopes (usually) or determinants and could be peptide epitopes (fragments of around 5-8 amino acids) or carbohydrate epitopes in the case of glycoproteins. If these epitopes are present in different species cross-reactivity may occur. The peptide epitopes could be linear or conformational. The conformational epitopes are more frequent and very variable because beside the variation of amino acids sequences are included into complex structural conformations of molecules. Usually, cross reactivity is encountered at proteins with at least 35% sequence similarity although the most phenomena of cross reactivity are meeting at the protein sequence identity greater than 50%, homologous proteins arises from a common origin, which share the same function, conserve the same overall folding and preserve the aspects of the core (double-stranded ß helices, α helices, ß-pleated sheets, and disulphide bridges). The loops of these proteins are more exposed, they present a lot of epitopes available for antibodies and able to participate in various evolutionary changes. However, it was shown that cross-reactivity can occur between non-homologous allergens [1].

In the allergic reaction process there are involved IgE, mast cells, basophils, and eosinophils which have different effects or functions. So, there must be at least two epitopes on the allergen molecule, with high affinity, which can bind two IgE molecules on the surface of mastocytes and basophils to activate those [2]. Therefore, when there are clinical phenomena of cross reaction that is associated with at least two allergens. A primary allergen is the original sensitizing molecule, it is the driving trigger and the secondary sensitization is due to cross-reactivity. In general, major allergens are also genuine and primary [3]. Cross reactivity between IgE and effector cells occurs when sequential similarity is more than 70% and very rarely when proteins have less than 50% sequence identity. Often a cross reactive allergen, named pan-allergen, belongs to a protein family well conserved throughout many widely different species. For example, members of the tropomyosin protein family, such as Der p 10 in house dust mite and Pen m 1 in black tiger shrimp [3]. Thus, taking these aspects into consideration, cross-reactivity should be analysed by evaluating both the taxonomic classification of organisms and the molecular classification of the allergens.

According to the taxonomic classification, peanut is a member of the legume family from Kingdom – Plantae, Order Fabales, Family – Fabaceae, Subfamily – Faboideae, tribe – Dalbergoeae, Genus Arachis, Species - *Arachis hypogaea*. Peanuts are very rich in nutrients and are one of the basic crops of India, China, the US and West Africa. The European Union (EU), Canada and

Japan import peanut mostly from the United States, Argentina, Sudan, Senegal, and Brazil.

According with the molecular classification the peanut allergens belong to the follow protein groups: Storage proteins (7S/11S globulins, 2S albumins, lectin superfamily: Ara h 1, Ara h 3, Ara h 2, Ara h 6; Ara h 7, Ara h agglutinin), Pathogenesis Related class 10 Protein (PR-10 proteins - Bet v-1-related proteins: Ara h 8), nsLTPs (non-specific Lipid Transfer Proteins: Ara h 9, Ara h 16, Ara h 17), Profilin family (Ara h 5), Oleosin family (Ara h 10, Ara h 11; Ara h 14, Ara h 15) and defensin family (Ara h 12, Ara h 13).

Thus, peanut allergens could cross-react on the one hand with the allergens from the same legume family and on the other hand with allergens from the other plant order or family but with the same ancestral origins like allergens from Pathogenesis Related class 10 Protein family or non-specific Lipid Transfer Proteins family.

In addition, it is clear that peanut allergens from different protein families could cross-react between them. A high cross reactivity is usually noticed between allergens from the same protein family from different plants and the allergenic reaction to a single peanut allergen is rarely. Indeed, it was shown that peanut allergic patients can be allergic to one or more legume or nuts too [1].

The number of protein types in peanut seed proteome are relatively low. But, some of the allergens have different isoforms, so, the proteomic investigation is quite difficult. Most studies on the phenomenon of cross reaction have been performed for the allergens Ara h 1, Ara h 2, Ara h 3 and Ara h 6. The content of all peanut allergens known up to date in peanut seed is around of 85% from total protein and Ara h 1, Ara h 2, and Ara h 3 accounting together for 75%.

The major peanut allergens Ara h 1, Ara h 2, and Ara h 3 are nonhomologous storage proteins as part of different food allergens family do not display linear sequence identities or structural similarities, nevertheless there is a high degree of IgE cross-reactivity among the 3 allergens. It was established that on the three allergens there are 3 groups of IgE epitopes: epitopes cross-reactive among all 3 allergens, epitopes unique for Ara h 2, and epitopes on Ara h 1, Ara h 3, or both not found on Ara h 2 but relevant only for a minority of patients. Withal, by cross-competitive ELISA assay it was showed that the affinity of IgE for Ara h 2 is higher than the affinity for Ara h 1 and Ara h 3. Additionally, Ara h 2 was more potent compared with Ara h 1 and Ara h 3 in basophil degranulation tests and skin prick tests and there were identified IgE binding peptides on Ara h 2 that are similar to peptides in Ara h 1 and Ara h 3

[13]. Although, Ara h 1 has a high concentration of 12-16% of the total protein of peanuts, the Ara h 2 is considered the most important peanut allergen, as it was identified as a predictor of clinical reactivity to peanut and is regarded as the most potent peanut allergen [5, 6, 7]. In a recently study it was observed that at the IgE level is an extensive cross-reactivity between Ara h 1, Ara h 2, Ara h 3 and Ara h 6 although with lower sensitizing than for the specific allergen. So, this study provide new and important information concerning cross-reactivity between some non-homologous peanut allergens [8].

Peanut allergens like Ara h 1, Ara h 2 and Ara h 3 have different cross-reactions with other allergens such as, those of soya bean, peas, lupine, fenugreek, lima beans, green beans, chickpeas, lentils or other beans but also with those of nuts [9].

Molecular modelling studies and clinical reports show that there is a structural basis for the cross-reactivity between Ara h 1, Len c 1 (lentil), Pis s 1 (pea), soya bean (Gly m 5) and with an allergen from lupine [7, 10].

Through the characterization of surface-exposed IgE-binding epitopes for the vicilin allergens of peanut (Ara h 1), walnut (Jug r 2), hazelnut (Cor a 11) and cashew nut (Ana o 1) it was showed that Ara h 1 cross - react these tree nuts allergens. In addition it was demonstrated that conformational epitopes (glyco-epitopes) corresponding to exposed *N*-glycosylation sites could also interfere with the IgE-binding epitopes, being susceptible to account for some cross-reactivity among the vicilin allergens [11]. Since 1981 it was considered that glycoproteins, like Ara h1, have carbohydrate epitopes, known as cross-reactive carbohydrate determinants (CCDs), may lead to the development of cross reactions between unrelated proteins, from very different sources such as plants and insects. For the carbohydrate determinants from Ara h 1 cross reactivity capacities were demonstrated [12] while for other peanut glycoproteins like Ara h 2, Ara h 3, Ara h 6 and Ara h 7 information on this topic are extremely scarce. In addition, the clinical relevance of CCD is still questioned and need more research.

Ara h 3 which is part of the same super family (Cupin superfamily) like Ara h 1, cross react with different allergens from nuts and also with allergens for example from spices like mustard. Thus, some studies showed that for Ara h 3 (peanut), Cor a 9 (hazelnut), Jug r 4 (walnut) and Ana o 2 (cashew nut) the surface-exposed IgE epitopes exhibited some structural similarities, thus accounting for the observed IgE cross-reactivity between peanut and tree nut allergens [13]. In addition the legumin-like Sin a 2 (mustard) has revealed IgE cross-reactivity with 11S globulins from peanut and tree nuts [14].

The peanut allergens of Prolamin superfamily - Conglutin family Ara h 2, Ara h 6 and Ara h 7 are 2S albumins. The conformational structures of Ara h 2 and Ara h 6 plays a critical role in allergenicity. The results of the immunological characterization of Ara h 2 and Ara h 6 provide evidence that, in addition to similar structural properties, these two peanut allergens share substantial cross-reactivity with regard to IgE antibody-binding capacity as well as in their allergenic potency, as shown by the results of the mediator-release experiments. Wild-type Ara h 2 and Ara h 6 have virtually identical allergenic potency as the allergens that were treated with digestive enzymes [15]. It has been demonstrated that at least parts of the Ara h 6 epitopes are cross-reactive with Ara h 2 epitopes although the first one is a minor allergen and the second one a major allergen [15, 16].

In addition, the major peanut allergen, Ara h 2, shares common IgE-binding epitopes with almond (Pru du 2S albumin) and Brazil nut (Ber e 1) allergens, which may contribute to the high incidence of tree nut sensitisation in peanut allergic individuals [17].

Other studies showed cross reactivity between Ara h 2 and the walnut vicilin Jug r 2 although these two allergens belong to different protein families and share only about 13% sequence identity [4, 7, 11, 18].

The cross reactivity between Ara h 1 and Ara h 2 and lupine major allergens α-, β- and δ-conglutin has been demonstrated. In the meantime, it seems that Ara h 3 and lupine γ-conglutin are involved in peanut-lupine cross reactivity into a much lesser extent [19].

Ara h 7 cross reactivity is not yet studied and presented in scientific papers.

Another group of peanut allergens which belong to Prolamin superfamily: Non-specific Lipid Transfer Protein family are represented by Ara h 9, Ara h 16 and Ara h 17. LTPs are highly conserved and widely distributed throughout the plant kingdom. Their biological function is to facilitate the transport of lipids, phospholipids and galacto-lipids across cellular membranes. LTPs are panallergens and strong cross-reactivity can be displayed among various plant food. Many studies have reported the importance of Ara h 9 in peanut-allergic patients. Ara h 9 shares 60-70% amino sequence identity with LTPs from a number of commonly consumed foods, including peach, apple, pear, plum, cherry, hazelnut, lentils, sunflower, beans, chestnut and strawberry. Other fruits and vegetables containing lipid transfer proteins that may result in cross-reactivity include sweet chestnut, cabbage, walnut, lettuce, pomegranate and hazelnut.

It was established that these allergens occupy a very important place in fruits from the Rosaceae (Prunoïdae). So, in those areas where Rosaceae fruits are widely consumed, in patients with peanut allergy, peach allergy should be considered a primary sensitization, and therefore testing Pru p 3 is recommended in those patients. In a study it was reported that ninety percent of 42 peanut-allergic patients were sensitized to Pru p 3, 82% to Ara h 9, and 74% to the hazelnut nsLTP Cor a 8. Pru p 3 showed a strong capacity to inhibit IgE-binding to Ara h 9 and Cor a 8, while Ara h 9 and Cor a 8 were unable to inhibit IgE-binding to Pru p 3 [20]. Allergenicity of fruit LTP depends on the occurrence of three IgE-binding epitopes at the surface of the proteins. According to this epitopic community, IgE-binding cross reactions frequently occur between LTP of different origin. Besides Rosaceae allergy, LTP are involved in many other food allergies and thus appear as particularly relevant food panallergens [21, 22].

Regarding Ara h 16 and Ara h 17, these allergens were just identified and are under provisionally accepted pending on IUIS meeting at EAACI 2015, respectively provisionally accepted, and will be voted on by IUIS at EAACI 2015. Currently, there are not enough data about these allergens and almost any clear data their implication in allergens cross reactivity.

Profilin family has only one representing of peanut, namely Ara h 5. This is a minor allergen with strong correspondence to other profilins of the birch tree and timothy grass pollen (Phl p 12 and Bet v 2), indicating cross-reactivity. Eight surface-exposed epitopes were found in Ara h 5 which, except some portions of epitopes 5 and 6, strongly coincided with the regions of validated linear epitopes in Bet v 2 (birch tree), Cuc m 2 (melon) and Hel a 2 (sunflower). Moreover, the epitopes #1, 5 and 7 are very similar relative to sequence and three dimensional conformations of profilins Ara h 5, Phl p 12, Bet v 2, Cuc m 2 and Hel a 2. All or some of these could be involved in cross reactivity. It should be noticed that Ara h 5 possess most epitopes among profilins [23]. Also, although sequence alignments show that Ara h 5 is more closely related to Hev b 8 (Hevea brasiliensis latex profilin), due to structure alignments Ara h 5 is more similar to Bet v 2 with some epitopes located at the loop regions and neutral to relatively electropositive sites on the protein surface, so more exposed and accessible [23, 24, 25].

Different profilin sensitization in peanut-allergic patients have been described in different areas of the world, with a sensitization rate of 3.3% in the United States, 9-16% in Northern and Central Europe, and 24% in Spanish peanut-allergic patients [7].

PR-10 (Pathogenesis Related class 10 Protein), Bet v-1-related proteins contains a peanut allergen namely Ara h 8. Through a lot of studies it was demonstrated that Bet v 1 from birch pollen often induces cross-reactive IgE with related allergens in certain fruits, vegetables, tree nuts and legumes including peanut. Thus, based on data that show a clinically relevant cross sensitization Hauser et al. grouped the family of Bet v 1 – related proteins into a Bet v 1 cluster which comprises allergens from a variety of different botanical sources: Aln g 1 (alder), Act c 8 (Kiwi), Api g 1 (celery), Gly m 4 (Soybean), Ara h 8 (peanut), Bet v 1 (birch pollen), Act d 8 (Kiwi), Dau c 1(carrot), Vig r 1 (mung bean), Cor a 1.04 (hazelnut), Car b 1 (carpinus), Cas s 1 (Sweet chestnut), Mal d 1 (apple), Cor a 1 (hazelnut), Pru ar 1 (Apricot), Fag s 1 (Beechnut), Pru av 1(cherry), Pru p 1 (peach), Pyr c 1 (pear), Que a 1 (White oak). These data showed that, and the risk to develop serious allergic reactions existed in individuals with concurrent birch pollen and peanut allergy [26].

The secondary structure similarities of Bet v 1 and Ara h 8 confirmed their ability to cross react. In addition, it was shown that the biologic activity of rAra h 8 was low compared with that of Bet v 1 or whole peanut extract. However, these observations strongly support the view that sensitization to the birch-related allergen Ara h 8 can cause clinical peanut allergy, including serious symptoms at least in a subgroup of sensitized patients [27]. The cross-reactivities between Bet v 1, Ara h 8 and Gly m 4 (the homolog from soya bean) and a potential cross reactivity with the specific protein from white lupine were confirmed [7, 28].

Peanut oleosins Ara h 10, Ara h 11; Ara h 14 and Ara h 15 have also been implicated in peanut hypersensitivity. For a while it was not clear whether peanut oil has or has not allergenicity [29, 30, 31]. Results of the studies were contradictory, but it was obvious that the allergenicity is affected by the refining process and the adverse reaction vary according to sensitive patient. Thus, a study shown that all protein are removed by an extensive process [32] but other showed that vegetable oils/fats, crude or even refined, can contain proteins - in peanut case peanut allergens - even that these were hot-pressed processed [33, 34, 35]. So, in the early 2000s it was suggested that peanut oil body-associated allergens such as oleosins are involved in allergic cross-reactivity to peanuts [36, 37]. Interestingly is that although, the first oleosins included in allergen database in 2001 were isoforms Ara h 14.0101 and Ara h 14.0102 with names Oleosin Variant A (currently has the accession number Q9AXI1_ARAHY) respectively Oleosin Variant B (currently has the accession number Q9AXI0_ARAHY). The most studied were the oleosins Ara h 10 and Ara h 11 which were included in allergen database in 2004 respectively 2005. The oleosins isoforms, at least the isoforms of allergen Ara h 14, do not only cross react by their central domains but also their N- and C-terminal domains [38, 39]. Although oleosins of peanuts are known for more than 10 years. There are very few studies on their allergenicity and possible cross reactivity. Pons et al. noticed a possible cross-reactivity between peanut and soya, based on their high sequence identity ranging from 50 to 79% [39]. Also Ara h 10 isoforms show a higher sequence identity to the hazelnut oleosin Cor a 12 (56%) and the sesame oleosin Ses i 4 (42%), while Ara h 11 shows higher sequence identity to Cor a 13 (69%) and Ses i 5 (75%) so it can be assumed that they are potential cross reactive [7]. Kobayashi et al. identified that a N-terminal part a peptide SDQTRTGY of Ara h 15.0101 (named in the paper Oleosin 3) is an IgE epitope which is responsible for cross-reactivity between peanut and buckwheat [40].

Peanut defensins Ara h 12 and Ara h 13 were included in allergen database recently (in 2012) and they do not have yet an access number in Uniprot database. Information about these proteins is extremely scarce. For example it is known that peanut defensins have very low sequence identity with defensins from other sources, so cross reactivity is not to be expected and IgE reactivity was shown for a small number of sera with severe peanut allergy.

Peanut lectin (Ara h agglutinin), considered a minor allergen can specifically interact with other closely related legume lectins like those from lentil, pea and kidney bean. These cross-reactivity is due of structurally related epitopes that have been identified on the molecular surface of these legume lectins. However, the clinical significance of the lectin-IgE interaction is not clearly clarified yet [41].

Some of the peanut allergenic molecules are glycoproteins, like Ara h 1 or Ara h agglutinin and it was reported that these allergens carrying one or more IgE-binding glycan side chains. The cross-reactive carbohydrate determinants (CCD) on the side chains of allergenic glycoproteins contribute to cross reactivity. Thus, the nonallergenic IgE-reactive glycoproteins in unrelated sources may influence and extend the pattern of CCD reactivity when allergenic extracts are tested and sometime the CCD-IgE co-recognition of similar carbohydrate structures on unrelated sources may lead to in vitro false positive results in diagnostic tests [42].

STABILITY AND MATRIX EFFECT

All proteins are polymers of amino acids, the sequence thereof is encoded by a gene. Each protein has its unique amino acid sequence determined from the nucleotide sequence of the gene. Secondary, tertiary and quaternary protein structure is carried out by weak interactions (like disulfide or hydrogen bonds) that can be broken even by changing the environmental conditions. An important external factor is the heat denaturation, increasing the temperature in a system lead to high molecular motion which then may lead to the breaking of hydrogen bonds. If these links are broken some structures become unstable, like α helices, resulting in weakness of the structure of proteins. In addition, food proteins are cleaved to amino acids in the hydrolytic action of proteolytic enzymes in the digestive juices (gastric pepsin, trypsin, chymotrypsin and carboxypeptidases intestinal juice, intestinal peptidases). Resulted amino acids are reabsorbed from the intestine through active mechanisms, moving in intestinal mucosal cells. Thus, being proteins, peanut allergens can suffer different modifications during food processing and digestion (acylation, polymerization, nitration, Maillard reaction, etc.), interactions within complex food matrices (both natural and fabricated structures). These modifications can reduce or increase their allergenic properties and are influenced by the food matrix.

Very important in the processing of peanuts is the place where are the epitopes. When epitopes are inside of the folded protein complex (conformational epitopes) it is possible that on cooking or processing food these epitopes to be modified so that allergenicity decrease or even be removed. If the epitopes are part of the continuous protein chain (linear epitopes) it is more likely that these to be more thermally stable. It is good to note that boiled peanuts appear to be less allergenic than those roasted. This phenomenon was observed in tropical Africa, China and Korea where, although consumption of boiled peanuts is widespread, allergy prevalence is lower compared to the US or Europe where peanuts are consumed mainly roasted and peanut allergy prevalence is high [43]. The diversity of food preparation has an important role in the prevalence of peanut allergy. It seems that the dry roasted peanuts are more allergic than boiled or fried peanuts but in the meantime cooking methods don't explain why the peanut allergy prevalence is lower in China matched up to Europe and America [32, 44, 45, 46, 47, 48, 49, 50].

The thermal processing of peanuts could also lead to new allergens through changing the shape of the protein and release of some "hidden" epitopes.

The allergenic globulins like Ara h 1 and Ara h 3 are generally less stable to thermal denaturation and enzymic digestion than nsLTPs or Ara h 8. However, it has been shown that the major peanut allergen, Ara h1, resists in most food processing method and is stable to digestion in the gastrointestinal tract. Ara h 1 purified heated at different temperatures although, shown a significant heat-induced denaturation on a molecular level, its IgE binding properties were similar to those of native Ara h 1, so the conformational epitopes seems to be protected by part of protein which are not sensitive to heat denaturation [51].

In the raw peanut, the structure of Ara h 1 is a trimeric complex in which potential cleavage sites for proteolytic digestion are inaccessible until the protein is denatured. By heat treatment, Ara h 1 becomes an aggregate with some epitopes destroyed but some of them have some protection from protease digestion and denaturation and allow passage of allergen across the small intestine. The highly stable nature of the Ara h 1 trimer, the presence of digestion resistant fragments, and the strategic location of the IgE-binding epitopes indicate that the quaternary structure of a protein may play a significant role in overall allergenicity [52, 53]. In addition, the intensity of heat treatment increase the hydrophobicity of Ara h 1 aggregates formed [54].

The bicupin core of Ara h 1 can be unfolded at low pH and reversibly folded at higher pH. Globulins aggregate at high temperature but also at low pH values. In these aggregates there are some partial α-helical structures and disulfide cross-links occur in relatively low amounts. The peptide fragments resulted from gastric digestion, in the basic environments, like the small intestine, become aggregates which protect and make epitopes available for triggering an allergic response [55].

The IgE-binding capacity of whole peanut extracts and purified the major peanut allergens Ara h 1 and Ara h 2 from raw, roasted and boiled peanuts was analyzed by the enzyme allergosorbent test (EAST) and EAST inhibition using the sera of peanut-allergic patients. As it was expected the composition of the peanut extracts was modified after heat processing, especially after boiling. It was shown that in boiled samples the low molecular allergens miss from the protein extracts but these proteins were found in the cooking water of peanuts. The IgE-binding capacity of boiled peanut extracts was tested on peanut sensitive patients. It was not observed any significant difference between protein extracts from raw and roasted peanuts. In the case of boiled samples The IgE-binding capacity was 2-fold lower than that of the extracts prepared from raw and roasted peanuts. It is very important to note that purified and roasted Ara h 1 and Ara h 2 had a higher IgE immunoreactivity compared with the same allergens in raw or boiled peanuts although, no significant difference in IgE binding capacity was observed between whole protein extracts from raw and roasted peanuts. According with these results it can be assumed that by roasting either hidden epitopes are exposed or new epitopes are provided, or both [56, 57]. In addition, it was demonstrated that Ara h 1 and especially Ara h 2 in the fried or roasted samples are more resistant to digestion with trypsin and pepsin than in the raw or boiled samples. Although, by trypsin or pepsin digestion for various periods of time, both allergens Ara h 1 and Ara h 2 in thermally processed samples are broken in numerous fragments (for example Ara h 1 in 84 fragments, and Ara h 2 in 21) quite a lot of fragments are capable of IgE binding, remaining allergenic for sensitive patients [58, 59]. The digestion of light roasted peanut, with other proteases like Alcalase or Flavourzyme, also showed a decreasing of Ara h 2 capacity to bind specific IgE [60].

A comparative analysis regarding the thermal resistance and to proteolysis of the major allergen Ara h 2 and the minor allergen Ara h 6, showed interesting results. The two allergens share substantial cross-reactivity, and are highly resistant to heat up to 100°C and to proteolytic digestion. Although, the reduction in IgE binding capacity was determined by heat and enzymatic treatments, the allergenic potency of both allergens were practically the same with the native Ara h 2 and Ara h 6. The explanation of this phenomenon resides in the fact that both allergens have virtually the same fold of the allergenic cores, the fold of the corresponding regions in the undigested proteins. The extreme immunological stability of the core structures of Ara h 2 and Ara h 6 provides an explanation for the persistence of the allergenic potency even after food processing [15].

Analysis of the effects of different autoclaving treatments applied to samples of raw, roasted, fried and boiled peanuts, have shown that the allergenicity is lost at different levels depending on the allergen and treatment. Thus, it was shown similar profiles of protein fragmentation after autoclaving treatments, especially after treatment at 138°C and 2.56 atm for 15 respectively 30 minutes. Especially allergens Ara h 1, Ara h 2 and Ara h 6 were analyzed. The usual autoclaving treatment (121°C, 1.18 atm, for 15 minutes) was less efficient in decreasing the allergens levels, but marked decrease in level of Ara h 2 and Ara h 6 was observed for all samples subjected to autoclaving more intense treatments. Instead, Ara h 1 was present in all the processed forms at different levels. Interestingly, in the basophil activation assay it was obtained a higher percentage of activation with boiled than with raw peanut but lower than with fried and roasted forms. It has been postulated that some neoallergens could be formed due to chemical modification during heating. However, it is clear that heat and pressure at specific conditions determine a decrease on the IgE binding properties and IgE cross-linking capacity of peanut proteins [61].

The enzymatic treatment in laboratory of Ara h 1 and Ara h 2 with digestive enzymes like α – chymotrypsin and trypsin, led to decrease in IgE -binding so it is possible that the enzymatic treatment has the potential to reduce the allergenicity of mentioned allergens, but clinical trials are necessary to confirm this reduction in allergenicity [62]. If before the enzymatic treatment, Ara h 1 and Ara h 2 from roasted peanuts are subjected to an ultrasound treatment is achieved a maximum reductions of allergens and lowest IgE binding [63].

In allergens which are glycoproteins, like Ara h 1, Ara h 2 and Ara h 3, in thermal process Maillard reactions could appear, meaning chemical reactions between amino acids (usually the ε-amino group of lysine residues) and reducing sugars. The reactive carbonyl group of the sugar reacts with the nucleophilic amino group of the amino acid, become glycosylated to form Amadori products, which degrade into dicarbonyl intermediates and forms a complex mixture of quite low characterized molecules, named *advanced glycation end products (AGE)*.

Dietary advanced glycation end products (AGEs) are known as glycotoxins, are a diverse group of highly oxidant compounds which could be implied besides allergenic properties in different diseases like diabetes, cardiovascular diseases, atherosclerosis, kidney disease oxidative stress, inflammation and in several other chronic diseases. In particular, broiling, roasting, and frying propagate and accelerate new AGE formation. The presence of reactive amino-lipids, as well as reducing sugars, such as fructose or glucose-6-phosphate, at heat treatments rapidly accelerates AGEs formation. In general, frying and roasting yielded more AGEs compared to boiling and steaming. Microwaving did not raise AGE content to the same extent as other dry heat cooking methods for the relatively short cooking times. For example, roasted peanuts have AGEs quantity (6,447 kU/100 g) higher than roasted beef (6,071 kU/100 g), similar to chicken breast roasted, 45 min with skin (6,639 kU/100 g) and much higher than other legumes [64].

In a study it was found AGE modifications on Ara h 1 and Ara h 3 in both raw and roasted peanut extract, and these compounds interacted with Receptor for AGE (RAGE) in dendritic cells of sensitive patients. At the same time, no AGE modifications and any RAGE interactions were found for Ara h 2. The mechanism of Maillard reaction is complex and involves numerous chemical rearrangements which finally lead to a lot of AGE products, some of them can have an impact on human health (hidden or new cross-reactive carbohydrate determinants epitopes – CCDs, acrylamide, heterocyclic amines – HCAs, glycation and lipoxidation end products). Like appearance, Maillard reaction leads to the occurrence of color compounds in various shades of brown, depending on the temperature and time at which takes place this process, with specific flavors. Actually, different studies showed that Ara h 1 and Ara h 2 subjected to thermal processing enhance the allergenic properties and bound higher levels of IgE, are more resistant to heat and digestion by gastrointestinal enzymes and Maillard reaction has a very important role to this [58, 65].

For example, the treatment of Ara h 1 at different time and temperatures with and without addition of glucose obviously shows different biochemical changes. Thus, at normal temperature of human body (37°C) with or without the addition of glucose, Maillard reactions are greatly reduced and pepsin hydrolysis is not limited. At 60°C Ara h 1 heated without glucose is degraded into low molecular weight protein fragments while at 145°C appear molecules with higher molecular weight than native one, therefore Maillard reactions are greatly reduced respectively in advanced stage. In the presence of additional glucose at 60°C appear products with molecular weight higher than of the native Ara h 1 (from 96 to 110 kDa) while at 145°C products with a range of molecular masses between 16 to 63.5kDa and the proportion of 63.5kDa is only 1.5%. In this situation Maillard reactions are in advanced stage for 60°C (light brown products) and final stage for 145°C (brown products) temperatures. Regarding the digestibility Ara h 1 after heating at the two temperatures significant differences occur. So, in absence of glucose the susceptibility to pepsin hydrolysis of Ara h 1 is not changed for both temperatures. When glucose added the degree of hydrolysis of Ara h 1 heated at 60°C increase while at 145°C decrease. It is worth to mention that raw Ara h 1 seems to have anti-proliferative actions on colon cancer cells and this characteristic is lost through Maillard reactions and pepsin hydrolysis [66, 67].

By synthesizing model peptides that imitate the model sequences which contain possible targets for glycation as well as the immunodominant epitopes of Ara h 2 and subjecting them to heat treatment, it was demonstrated that overlapping major epitopes 6 and 7, which do not contain any lysine or arginine moieties, it obtained a higher level of IgE binding when subjected to Maillard reaction. So, it was established that nonbasic amino acids might be accessible for nonenzymatic glycation reactions and that these posttranslational modifications might induce increased IgE binding of the glycated Ara h 2. Similar experiments with peanut agglutinin, considered a minor allergen, showed that after heat treatment appear at peanut-sensitive patients a high level of IgE binding to the lectin [68].

It was demonstrated that allergenic properties of peanut allergens could be reduced when in matrix are present polyphenols, phenols (for example caffeic acid) and/or polyphenol oxidase or peroxidase. These enzymes catalyzes the oxidation of tyrosine residues of proteins and, therefore, their cross-linking led to a reduction of the allergenic properties. For example, polyphenol oxidase/caffeic acid reduced the allergenic properties of Ara h 1 and Ara h 2 by cross-linking and decreasing the levels of allergens [69].

A study showed that peanut allergens Ara h 2 and Ara h 3 cranberry or green tea polyphenol complexes are more rapidly hydrolysed by pepsin compared to uncomplexed allergens and protein fragments obtained had substantially lower capacity to bind to peanut-specific IgE of sensitive patients as compared with the peptides from uncomplexed peanut flour. So, the presence in the matrix of phenols reduce the allergenicity of peanut allergens in peanuts for example of Ara h 2 and Ara h 3 [70].

The non-specific Lipid Transfer Proteins constitutes a group of proteins stable to heat and digestion, causing reactions even in processed food. The four conserved disulfide bridges linking different regions of the polypeptide chain make Lipid transfer proteins (LTP) extremely resistant to both heat denaturation (cooking) and proteolysis by digestive enzymes. Such a resistance to denaturation significantly account for their allergenicity [21]. Due to its stability to food processing and resistance to proteolytic digestion, it has been proposed that LTP may reach the intestinal tract in an almost unmodified form [71, 72].

The IgE reactivity and the proteolytic stability of native Ara h 8 was shown to be increased after roasting possibly due to the association of the allergen with lipophilic ligands and/or the formation of neo-epitopes. Among potential ligands with strong binding capacity in the hydrophobic cavity of Ara h 8.0101 have been identified the phytoestrogen flavonoids quercetin, apigenin, and daidzein, suggesting that Ara h 8 might serve as a delivery vehicle for flavonoids. The gastric digestion experiments demonstrated low proteolytic stability of recombinant Ara h 8, whereas the stability of native Ara h 8 was increasingly higher in unroasted and roasted peanut. This stability is probably due to Maillard reactions, lipid oxidations, and lipophilic associations [7, 73].

The differences or even discrepancies between results of different authors can be attributed to different methods of experimentation, such as protein extraction, purification, glycation, temperatures of heating, etc.

It seems that matrixes with polyphenols, phenols (for example caffeic acid) and/or polyphenol oxidase or peroxidase decrease the peanut allergens level.

As a general conclusion it can be said that more detailed research are needed to clearly determine what the transformations are which allergens suffer to different types of cooking and matrixes, in order to find some precise means to decrease the allergenicity of peanuts.

REFERENCES

[1]   Sicherer, S.H., Wood, R.A., the Section on Allergy and Immunology. (2012). Allergy testing in childhood: using allergen-specific IgE tests. *Pediatrics,* 129(1), 193-197.

[2]   Stone, K.D., Prussin, C., Metcalfe, D.D., (2010). IgE, Mast Cells, Basophils, and Eosinophils. *The Journal of Allergy and Clinical Immunology*, 125(2 Suppl. 2), S73-S80.

[3]   Canonica, G.W., Ansotegui, I.J., Pawankar, R., Schmid-Grendelmeier, P., van Hage, M., Baena-Cagnani, C.E., Melioli, G., Nunes, C., Passalacqua, G., Rosenwasser, L., Sampson, H., Sastre, J., (2013). A WAO - ARIA - GA2LEN consensus document on molecular-based allergy diagnostics. *World Allergy Organization Journal*, 6:17.

[4]   Bublin, M., Kostadinova, M., Radauer, C., Hafner, C., Szépfalusi, Z., Varga, E-M., Maleki, S.J., Hoffmann-Sommergruber, K., Breiteneder, H., (2013). IgE cross-reactivity between the major peanut allergen Ara h 2 and the nonhomologous allergens Ara h 1 and Ara h 3. *J Allergy Clin Immunol*. 132, 118-24.

[5]   Koppelman, S.J., Wensing, M., Ertmann, M., Knulst, A.C., Knol, E.F., (2004). Relevance of Ara h 1, Ara h 2 and Ara h 3 in peanut-allergic patients, as determined by immunoglobulin E Western blotting, basophil-histamine release and intracutaneous testing: Ara h 2 is the most important peanut allergen. *Clin. Exp. Allergy* 34, 583-590.

[6]   Lin, J., Bruni, F.M., Fu, Z.Y., Maloney, J., Bardina, L., Boner, A.L., Gimenez, G., Sampson, H.A., (2012). A bioinformatics approach to identify patients with symptomatic peanut allergy using peptide microarray immunoassay. *J Allergy Clin Immunol.*, 129(5), 1321-1328. e5.

[7]   Bublin, M., Breiteneder, H., (2014). Cross-Reactivity of Peanut Allergens. *Curr Allergy Asthma Rep*. 14(4): 426.

[8] Smit, J.J., Pennings, M.T., Willemsen, K., van Roest, M., van Hoffen, E., Pieters, R.H., (2015). Heterogeneous responses and cross reactivity between the major peanut allergens Ara h 1, 2, 3 and 6 in a mouse model for peanut allergy. *Clinical and Translational Allergy*. 5: 13.

[9] Fæste, C.K., Namork, E., (2010). Differentiated Patterns of Legume Sensitisation in Peanut-Allergic Patients. *Food Anal. Methods*. 3, 357-362.

[10] Chruszcz, M., Maleki, S.J., Majorek, K.A., Demas, M., Bublin, M., Solberg, R., Hurlburt, B.K., Ruan, S., Mattisohn, C.P., Breiteneder, H., Minor, W., (2011). Structural and Immunologic Characterization of Ara h 1, a Major Peanut Allergen. *The Journal of Biological Chemistry*. 286 (45), 39318-39327.

[11] Barre, A., Sordet, C., Culerrier, R., Rancé, F., Didier, A., Rougé, P., (2008). Vicilin allergens of peanut and tree nuts (walnut, hazelnut and cashew nut) share structurally related IgE-binding epitopes. *Mol. Immunol*. 45, 1231-1240.

[12] Mueller, G.A., Maleki, S.J., Johnson, K., Hurlburt, B.K., Cheng, H., Ruan, S., Nesbit, J.B., Pomés, A., Edwards, L.L., Schorzman, A., Deterding, L.J., Park, H., Tomer, K.B., London, R.E., Williams, J.G., (2013). Identification of Maillard reaction products on peanut allergens that influence binding to the receptor for advanced glycation end products. *Allergy*. 68(12), 1546-1554.

[13] Barre, A., Jacquet, G., Sordet, C., Culerrier, R., Rouge, P., (2007). Homology modelling and conformational analysis of IgE-binding epitopes of Ara h 3 and other legumin allergens with a cupin fold from tree nuts. *Mol Immunol*. 44(12), 3243-3255.

[14] Sirvent S, Akotenou M, Cuesta-Herranz J, Vereda A, Rodriguez, R, Villalba M, Palomares, O., (2012). The 11S globulin Sin a 2 from yellow mustard seeds shows IgE cross-reactivity with homologous counterparts from tree nuts and peanut. *Clin Transl Allergy*. 2(1), 23.

[15] Lehmann, K., Schweimer, K., Reese, G., Randow, S., Suhr, M., Becker, W. M., Vieths, S., Rosch, P., (2006). Structure and stability of 2S albumin-type peanut allergens: implications for the severity of peanut allergic reactions. *Biochem J*. 395(3), 463-472.

[16] Schmidt, H., Gelhaus, C., Latendorf, T., Nebendahl, M., Petersen, A., Krause, S., Leippe, M., Becker, W. M., Janssen, O., (2009). 2-D DIGE analysis of the proteome of extracts from peanut variants reveals striking differences in major allergen contents. *Proteomics*. 9, 3507-3521.

[17] de Leon, M.P., Drew,A.C., Glaspole, I.N., Suphioglu, C., O'Hehir, R.E., Rolland, J.M., (2007). IgE cross-reactivity between the major peanut allergen Ara h 2 and tree nut allergens. *Molecular Immunology.* 44, 463-471.

[18] Maleki, S.J., Bublin, M., Chruszcz, M., Charles, T., Grimm, C.C., Cheng, H., Teuber, S.S., Hurlburt, B.K., Breiteneder, H., Schein, C., (2015). Identification of the epitopes that cause cross-reactions between peanuts and tree nuts. *Journal of Allergy and Clinical Immunology.* 135 (2), Supplement, pp.AB32.

[19] Dooper, M.M.B.W., Plassen, C., Holden, L., Lindvik, H., Fæste, C.K., (2009). Immunoglobulin E Cross-Reactivity between Lupine Conglutins and Peanut Allergens in Serum of Lupine-Allergic Individuals. *J Investig Allergol Clin Immunol* 19(4), 283-291.

[20] Javaloyes G, Goikoetxea MJ, Garcia Nunez I, Aranda A, Sanz ML, Blanca M, Diaz-Perales, A., da Souza, J., Esparza, I., delPozo, V., Blazquez, A.B., Sceurer, S., Vieths, S., Ferrer, M., (2012). Pru p 3 acts as a strong sensitizer for peanut allergy in Spain. *J Allergy Clin. Immunol.* 130(6), 1432-1434.

[21] Rouge, P., Borges, J-P., Culerrier, R., Brule, C., Didier, A. Barre, A., (2009). Les proteines de transfert des lipides: des allergenes importants des fruits. *Revue française d'allergologie* 49, 58-61.

[22] Romano, A., Fernandez-Rivas, M. Caringi, M., Amato, S., Mistrello, G., Asero, R., (2009). Allergy to peanut lipid transfer protein (LTP): frequency and cross-reactivity between peanut and peach LTP. *Eur Ann Allergy Clin Immunol.* 41(4), 106-111.

[23] Cabanos, C., Tandang-Silvas, M. R., Odijk, V., Brostedt, P., Tanaka, A., Utsumi, S., and Maruyama, N., (2010). Expression, purification, cross-reactivity and homology modeling of peanut profilin. *Protein Expr Purif.* 73(1), 36-45.

[24] Wang, Y., Fu, T. J., Howard, A., Kothary, M. H., McHugh, T. H., Zhang, Y., (2013). Crystal structure of peanut (Arachis hypogaea) allergen Ara h 5. *J Agric Food Chem.* 61(7), 1573-1578.

[25] García, B.E., Lizaso, M.T., (2011). Cross-reactivity Syndromes in Food Allergy. *J Investig Allergol Clin Immunol.* 21(3), 162-170.

[26] Hauser, M., Roulias, A., Ferreira, F., Egger, M., (2010). Panallergens and their impact on the allergic patient. *Allergy Asthma Clin Immunol.* 6 (1), 1.

[27] Mittag D, Akkerdaas J, Ballmer-Weber BK, Vogel L, Wensing M, Becker WM, Koppelman, S.J., Knulst, A.C., Helbling, A., Hefle, S.L., van Ree,

R., Vieths, S., (2004). Ara h 8, a Bet v 1-homologous allergen from peanut, is a major allergen in patients with combined birch pollen and peanut allergy. *J Allergy Clin Immunol.* 114(6):1410-1417.

[28] Hurlburt, B. K., Offermann, L. R., McBride, J. K., Majorek, K. A., Maleki, S. J., Chruszcz, M., (2013). Structure and function of the peanut panallergen Ara h 8. *J Biol Chem.* 288(52), 36890-36901.

[29] Moneret-Vautrin, D.A., Hatahet, R., Kanny, G., Ait-Djafer, Z., (1991). Allergenic peanut oil in milk formulas. *The Lancet.* 338(8775): 1149.

[30] Moneret-Vautrin, D.A., Hatahet, R., Kanny, G., (1994). Risks of milk formulas containing peanut oil contaminated with peanut allergens in infants with atopic dermatitis. *Pediatr Allergy Immunol.* 5(3): 184-188.

[31] Hourihane, J.O., Bedwani, S.J. Dean, T.P., Warner, J.O., (1997). Randomised, double blind, crossover challenge study of allergenicity of peanut oils in subjects allergic to peanuts. *BMJ.* 314(7087), 1084-1088.

[32] Hefle, S.L., (1999). Impact of processing on food allergens. *Adv Exp Med Biol.* 459, 107-109.

[33] Klurfeld, D.M., Kritchevsky, D., (1987). Isolation and quantitation of lectins from vegetable oils. *Lipids.* 22(9), 667-668.

[34] Teuber, S.S., Brown, R.L., Haapanen, L.A., (1997). Allergenicity of gourmet nut oils processed by different methods. *J Allergy Clin Immunol.* 99(4), 502-507.

[35] Hidalgo, F.J., Alaiz, M., Zamora, M., (2001). Determination of peptides and proteins in fats and oils. *Anal Chem.* 73(3), 698-702.

[36] Pons, L., Olszewski, A., Guéant, J.L., (1998). Characterization of the oligomeric behavior of a 16.5 kDa peanut oleosin by chromatography and electrophoresis of the iodinated form. *J Chromatogr B Biomed Sci Appl.* 706(1), 131-140.

[37] Pons, L., Chery, C., Romano, A., Namour, F., Artesani, M. C., Gueant, J.L., (2002). The 18 kDa peanut oleosin is a candidate allergen for IgE-mediated reactions to peanuts. *Allergy.* 57 Suppl. 72, 88-93.

[38] http://www.allergen.org.

[39] Pons, L., Chery, C., Mrabet, N., Schohn, H., Lapicque, F., Gueant, J.L., (2005). Purification and cloning of two high molecular mass isoforms of peanut seed oleosin encoded by cDNAs of equal sizes. *Plant Physiol Biochem.* 43(7), 659-668.

[40] Kobayashi, S., Katsuyama, S., Wagatsuma, T., Okada, S., Tanabe, S., (2012). Identification of a new IgEbinding epitope of peanut oleosin that cross-reacts with buckwheat. *Biosci Biotechnol Biochem.* 76(6), 1182-1188.

[41] Rouge, P., Culerrier, R., Granier, C., Rance, F., Barre, A., (2010). Characterization of IgE-binding epitopes of peanut (Arachis hypogaea) PNA lectin allergen cross-reacting with other structurally related legume lectins. *Mol Immunol.* 47(14), 2359-2366.

[42] Ferreira, F., Hawranek, T., Gruber, P., Wopfner, N., Mari, A., (2004). Allergic cross-reactivity: from gene to the clinic. *Allergy.* 59, 243-267.

[43] Jackson, W.F. (2003). Food Allergy – ILSI Europe concise monograph series. http://europe.ilsi.org/publications.

[44] Sampson, H.A., (2004). Update on food allergy. *J Allergy Clin Immunol.* 113(5), 805-819.

[45] Chung, S.Y., Butts, C.L. Maleki, S.J., Champagne, E.T., (2003). Linking peanut allergenicity to the processes of maturation, curing, and roasting. *J Agric Food Chem.* 51(15), 4273-4277.

[46] Sathe, S.K., Sharma, G.M., (2009). Effects of food processing on food allergens. *Molecular Nutrition and Food Research.* 53(8), 970-978.

[47] Poms, R.E., Anklam, E., (2004). Effects of chemical, physical, and technological processes on the nature of food allergens. *J AOAC Int.* 87 (6), 1466-1474.

[48] Maleki, S.J., Viquez, O., Jacks, T., Dodo, H., Champagne, E.T., Chung, S-Y., Landry, S.J., (2003). The major peanut allergen, Ara h 2, functions as a trypsin inhibitor, and roasting enhances this function. *J Allergy Clin Immunol.* 112(1), 190-195.

[49] Kopper, R. A., N. J. Odum, Sen, M., Helm, R.M., Stanley, J.S., Burks, A.W., (2005). Peanut protein allergens: the effect of roasting on solubility and allergenicity. *Int Arch Allergy Immunol.* 136(1), 16-22.

[50] Cong, Y-J., Lou, F., Xue, W-T., Li, L-F, Wang, J., Zhang, H., (2007). The effect of cooking methods on the allergenicity of peanut. *Food and Agricultural Immunology.* 18(1), 53-65.

[51] Koppelman, S.J., Bruijnzeel-Koomen, C.A., Hessing, M., de Jongh, H.H., (1999). Heat-induced conformational changes of Ara h 1, a major peanut allergen, do not affect its allergenic properties. *J Biol Chem.* 274 (8), 4770-4777.

[52] Maleki, S.J., Kopper, R.A., Shin, D.S., Park, C.W., Compadre, C.M., Sampson, H., Burks, A.W., Bannon, G.A., (2000). Structure of the major peanut allergen Ara h 1 may protect IgE-binding epitopes from degradation. *J Immunol.* 164(11), 5844-5849.

[53] Shin, D.S., Compadre, C.M., Maleki, S.J., Kopper, R.A., Sampson, H., Huang, S.K., Burks, A.W., Bannon, G.A., (1998). Biochemical and structural analysis of the IgE binding sites on Ara h1, an abundant and

highly allergenic peanut protein. *The Journal of Biological Chemistry*. 273(22), 13753-13759.

[54] Montserrat, M., Mayayo, C., Sánchez, L., Calvo, M., Pérez, M.D., (2013). Study of the thermoresistance of the allergenic Ara h 1protein from peanut (Arachis hypogaea). *J.Agric.Food Chem*. 61(13), 3335-3340.

[55] Khan, I.J., Di, R., Patel, P., Nanda, V., (2013). Evaluating disulfide crosslinking and pH-induced aggregation of Arachis hypogea 1 as components of Peanut Allergy. *J Agric Food Chem*. 61(35), 8430–8435.

[56] Maleki, S.J., Viquez, O., Jacks, T., Dodo, H., Champagne, E.T., Chung, S.Y., Landry, S.J., (2003). The major peanut allergen, Ara h 2, functions as a trypsin inhibitor, and roasting enhances this function. *J Allergy Clin Immunol*. 112(1), 190-195.

[57] Mondoulet, L., Paty, E., Drumare, M.F., Ah-Leung, S., Scheinmann, P., Willemot, R.M., Wal, J.M., Bernard, H., (2005). Influence of Thermal Processing on the Allergenicity of Peanut Proteins. *J. Agric. Food Chem*. 53(11), 4547-4553.

[58] Maleki, S.J., Schmitt, D.A., Galeano, M., Hurlburt, B.K., (2014). Comparison of the Digestibility of the Major Peanut Allergens in Thermally Processed Peanuts and in Pure Form. *Foods*. 3, 290-303.

[59] Vissers, Y.M., Blanc, F., Skov, P.S., Johnson, P.E., Rigby, N.M., Przybylski-Nicaise, L., Bernard, H., Wal, J.M., Ballmer-Weber, B., Zuidmeer-Jongejan, L., Szepfalusi, Z., Ruinemans-Koerts, J., Jansen, A.P., Savelkoul, H.F., Wichers, H.J., Mackie, A.R., Mills, C.E., Adel-Patient, K., (2011). Effect of heating and glycation on the allergenicity of 2S albumins (Ara h 2/6) from peanut. *PLoS One*. 6(8), e23998.

[60] Shi, X., Guo, R., White, B.L., Yancey, A., Sanders, T.H., Davis, J.P., Burks, A.W., Kulis, M., (2013). Allergenic properties of enzymatically hydrolysed peanut flour extracts. *Int Arch Allergy Immunol*. 162(2), 123-130.

[61] Cabanillas, B., Cuadrado, C., Rodriguez, J., Hart, J., Burbano, C., Crespo, J.F., Novak, N., (2015). Potential changes in the allergenicity of three forms of peanut after thermal processing. *Food Chemistry*. 183, 18-25.

[62] Yu, J., Goktepe, I., Ahmedna, M., (2013). Enzymatic treatment of peanut butter to reduce the concentration of major peanut allergens. *Int. J. Food Sci. Technol*. 48(6), 1224-1234.

[63] Li, H., Yu, J., Ahmedna, M., Goktepe, I., (2013). Reduction of major peanut allergens Ara h 1 and Ara h 2, in roasted peanuts by ultrasound assisted enzymatic treatment. *Food Chem*. 141(2), 762-768.

Chapter 4

METHODS FOR DETECTING, QUANTIFYING AND CHARACTERISING PEANUT ALLERGENS

Maria Pele, PhD**[*] **and Carmen Cimpeanu, PhD
University of Agronomic Sciences and Veterinary Medicine Bucharest,
Bucharest, Romania

ABSTRACT

The commonly used methods for identifying, quantifying and characterising the major peanut allergens in food are mainly immunochemical and molecular. The most used method to identify peanut allergens in different foods are ELISA and dipstick. However, in the last twenty years there have been developed methods based on SDS-PAGE, HPLC techniques coupled or not with mass spectrometry, capillary electrophoresis, circular dichroism, FTIR, NMR, X-ray spectroscopy or immunochemical sensors. Nevertheless, studies on peanut allergens using these methods are quite few. It has to specify that for the establishment of peanut allergens crystal structure X-ray spectrometry was mainly used. This review focuses on the articles appeared up-to-date concerning alternative methods to quantify allergens to those based on immunochemical or molecular evaluations.

---

[*] Corresponding author: Maria Pele. Email: mpele50@yahoo.com.

Keywords: peanut allergens, identification, quantification, characterization

INTRODUCTION

Proteomics, analysis and characterization of proteome, has nowadays a development comparable with those of genomics in 1990s. Since the human genome sequence has been established in 2000, the determination of structure, expression and function of all proteins has become a huge task for researchers. If in a cell there are around 30-40 thousands of gene the number of proteins and peptides is at level of several hundreds of thousands. Because of continuous changes in the cell at the proteome level, proteins and peptides are in different forms and functions and varies in time so a protein can exist in cell at a certain time and disappear in other or becomes different after posttranslational modifications like phosphorylation, glycosylation, oxidation, etc. Moreover the protein content of cells varies widely even if each cell is a given organism containing the same genome. This kind of complexity could make difficult the identification, characterisation and quantitative determination of proteins. However the knowledge about proteins has increased in last decade even if we take into account only the number (several thousands) of publications which appear each year containing the terms "proteome" or "proteomics."

Peanut shares many cross-reacting proteins with other members of Leguminous family and this makes more difficult the task to detect low quantities of it in food.

The presence of other abundant proteins can mask low abundance proteins especially in food like cookies, chocolates, sauces, etc. where the matrix is complex.

There is no doubt that the useful methods for allergen characterisation are complex, as allergen characterization is a difficult and troublesome task.

Nevertheless, food allergies have been established as major risk issues that the food industry can no longer ignore. Allergen labelling regulations oblige the companies to label all pre-packed food if they contain any of the listed allergenic components as an ingredient (Australia – 10, Canada – 11, China – 9, EU – 14, Japan – 5, Korea – 7, Mexico – 8, South Africa – 9, US - 8) [1]. In order to check the presence of allergens in food, the food industry has the possibility to use commercial kits available on market. The common methods used to quantitative or semi-quantitative detect the allergens (peanut allergens) are immunological or molecular methods like ELISA and PCR. The amount and quality of published data from objective sources regarding the analysis methodologies used to characterise the peanut allergens varies remarkably.

Regarding the methods used for protein/allergens separation, identification, characterisation and quantification there are a lot of papers published in the last 20 years in which a large number of different methods are described.

The published papers showed that the most modern methods used until now, besides ELISA and PCR methods, for separation, identification, characterization and monitoring biological activity of proteins/allergens belongs to three big analytical chemistry fields: electrochemistry (electrophoresis, capillary electrophoresis), chromatography (Gel Chromatography, HPLC, LC, etc.) and spectrophotometry (Circular Dichroism, Mass Spectrophotometry, NMR).

Most researchers usually use tandem methods from at least two chemistry fields. There are very few papers which presents only one kind of methods.

Even there are few reports regarding quantitative determination of peanut or other allergens by other specific methods than immunological or molecular ones, it doesn't mean that the alternative methods are not useful at all, on the contrary.

The aim of the present review in this context is to have a general view about the alternative methods for allergens quantification and specifically for peanut allergens.

A general pathway for separation, identification, characterization, detection and quantification of proteins/allergens is to collect the sample, to handle and storage it, to separate the protein/allergen, to purify, concentrate, identify, characterize, quantify and results publication. The most studies concerning allergens use different methods, some of them in tandem, to identify, quantify and characterise them. The most used methods to analyse protein allergens are represented in Figure 1. It has to be highlighted the fact that there are extremely few studies which used only one kind of analytical method.

Innovative analytical methods and novel applications of available techniques are required to deal with the food allergenicity problems in an integrated manner.

IMMUNOCHEMICAL AND MOLECULAR METHODS

Peanut allergens in different food are usually detected by immunological or molecular methods like ELISA and PCR. All immunochemical techniques use a specific antibody (polyclonal or monoclonal) and the PCR methods need specific DNA fragments so that it is necessary a separate analysis for each allergen present in food. Nowadays there are competitive commercial available ELISAs and DNA-based test kits for allergen detection in food products, but only a few of them are validated by inter-laboratory studies. at this time there is also a small quantity of information and published data available concerning commercially available dipstick [2-7]. Immunochemical techniques for the analysis of proteins, based on immunological principles, which have been proved adequate for the specific detection of allergens in food are radio-allergosorbent assay (RAST), radioimmuno assay (RIA), rocket immunoelectrophoresis (RIE), enzyme-allergosorbent tests (EAST), immunoblotting and enzyme-linked immunosorbent assays (ELISA). Using of rocket immunoelectrophoresis, made possible the determination of amounts of 10 ppm even for the smallest of peanut proteins especially in chocolates but the classical RAST, RIE and RIA need, specific antibodies, namely patients sera which are not easily available [8].

With the development of methods for obtaining the polyclonal and monoclonal antibodies, different methods based on Enzyme Linked Immunosorbents Assay (ELISA) have been achieved. ELISA methods (direct, indirect, sandwich, competitive or inhibition) detect the allergen protein molecules by binding antibodies to the allergen and then using an enzyme-linked conjugate to create a colorimetric change that can be spectro-photometrically measured.

The development of genomics and the possibility of establishing specific genes for making proteins were performed by techniques based on polymerase chain reaction (PCR). PCR methods (PCR, real-time PCR or quantitative PCR, Reverse transcription polymerase chain reaction, Real-Time Quantitative Reverse Transcription PCR), typically amplifies DNA fragments of the allergens which must be identified or quantified. The amount of amplified products is determined by the available substrates in the reaction, which become limited as the reaction progresses. These methods are more sensitive ones and can be used in raw and cooked products and are not affected by the heating process because DNA typically remains intact after being exposed to the cooking temperatures of most foods and are not subject to the typical interferences specific to ELISA methods. However, PCR methods cannot be used for products which do not contain DNA, such as peanut oil [9].

Some of the currently available commercial peanut test kits are summarized in Table 1.

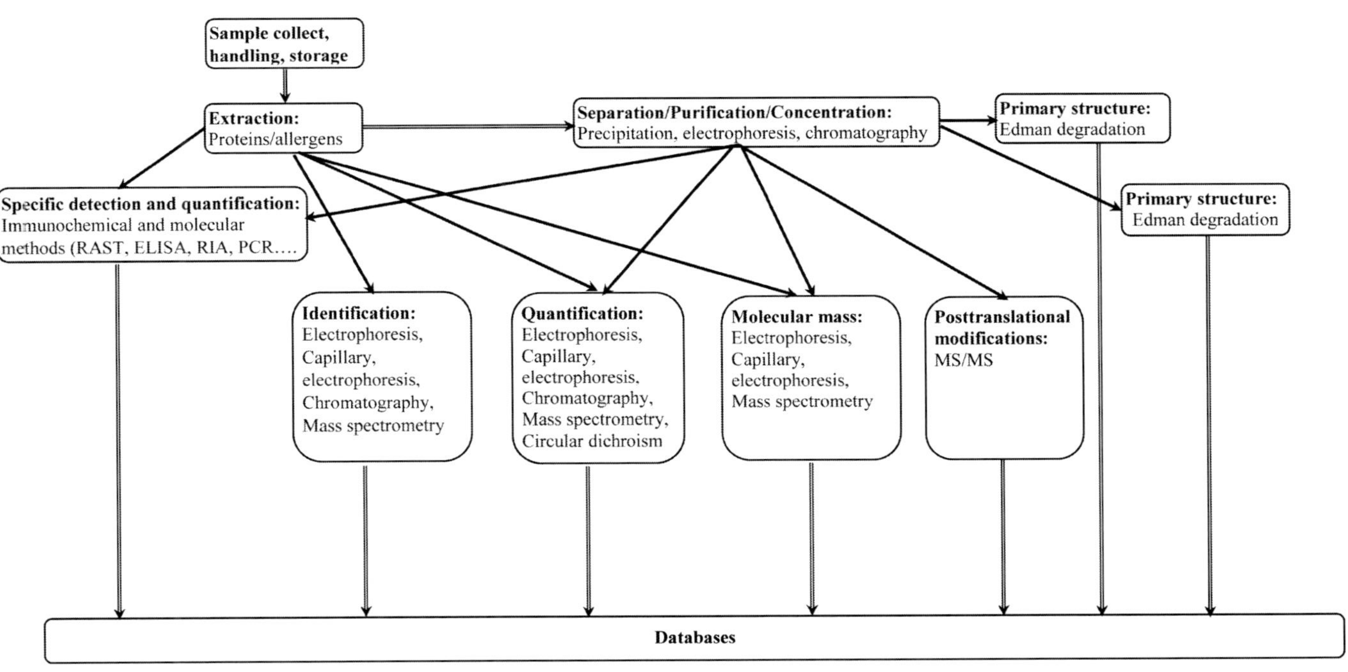

Figure 1. Diagram representing the most used methods for chemical and biochemical characterisation of allergens.

Table 1. The main currently available peanut test kits

Company	Kits	Type	LOD[a]	LOQ[b]
Protein based methods				
Bio-Check (UK)	Peanut-Check Kit	Quantitative ELISA Technique	0.13 ppm	0.25 ppm
BioFront Technologies	Peanut Protein ELISA Kit	Quantitative ELISA Technique	0.3 ppm	1 ppm
R-Biopharm	Lateral Flow Peanut	Qualitative Lateral Flow Device	1 ppm	
R-Biopharm	RIDASCREEN FAST Peanut	Quantitative ELISA Technique	1.5 ppm	2.5 ppm
Crystal Chem	Peanut ELISA Kit	Quantitative ELISA Technique	0.3 ppm	0.78 ppm
ELISA-Systems	ELISA Systems Peanut *Ara h 1* and *Ara h 2*	Quantitative ELISA Technique	1 ppm	2.5 ppm
ELUTION Technologies	Peanut Protein Rapid Test	Qualitative Lateral Flow Device	2 ppm	
ELUTION Technologies	Peanut Protein ELISA Kit	Quantitative ELISA Technique	2 ppm	2 ppm
Hygiena	AllerSnap Allergen Prevention Kit from	Qualitative Lateral Flow Device	2 ppm	
INDOOR Biotechnologies	Ara h 1 ELISA kit (EL-AH1)	Qualitative	31.5 ng/ml	-
INDOOR Biotechnologies	Ara h 2 ELISA kit (EL-AH2)	Qualitative	2 ng/ml	-
INDOOR Biotechnologies	Ara h 6 ELISA kit (EL-AH6)	Qualitative	0.8 ng/ml	-
Morinaga Institute of Biological Science, Inc.	Lateral Flow Peanut	Qualitative Lateral Flow Device	5 ppm	

Table 1. (Continued)

Company	Kits	Type	LOD[a]	LOQ[b]
Neogen	Reveal 3-D Peanut	Qualitative Lateral Flow Device	5 ppm	-
Neogen	Reveal Peanut	Qualitative Lateral Flow Device	5 ppm	-
Neogen	BioKits Peanut	Quantitative ELISA Technique	0.1 ppm	1 ppm
Neogen	Veratox Peanut	Quantitative ELISA Technique	1 ppm	2.5 ppm
Romer Labs	AgriStrip Peanut	Qualitative Lateral Flow Device	1 ppm	-
Romer Labs	Agra Quant Peanut	Quantitative ELISA Technique	0.1 ppm	2 ppm
Romer Labs	Agra Quant Plus Peanut	Quantitative ELISA Technique	0.5 ppm	2 ppm
Tecna Lab	I'Screen Peanut	Quantitative ELISA Technique	1.6 ppm	1.6 ppm
DNA based methods				
R-Biopharm	SureFood ALLERGEN Peanut	Qualitative RT-PCR Technique	<1 mg/kg	-
R-Biopharm	SureFood QUNAT Peanut	Quantitative RT-PCR Technique	<1 mg/kg	4 mg/kg
R-Biopharm	SureFood ALLERGEN 4 Plex Peanut/Hazelnut/ Walnut + IAC	Qualitative RT-PCR Technique	<1 mg/kg	-
Neogen	BioKits Peanut	Qualitative RT-PCR Technique	<1 mg/kg	-

[a] LOD = Limit of detection.

[b] LOQ = Limit of quantification.

In the last twenty years, various companies have developed the production of kits for the determination of peanut protein and the majority of them are using sandwich ELISA techniques for qualitative or quantitative determinations. The limits of detection and the limits for quantification specified by the manufacturers widely vary in a range of 0.04-5 ppm respectively 1-40 ppm. The majority of kits are designed for the detection and/or quantification of peanut proteins.

The lateral flow devices are designed to show in a short time if the analyzed food contain or not peanut traces. These are cheap and portable kits without any other required equipment.

Some companies like INDOOR biotechnologies have been achieved specific kits for peanuts allergens such as Ara h 1, Ara h 2 and Ara h 6 or ELISA Systems and R-Biopharm for Ara h 1 and Ara h 2.

The PCR based kits are extremely accurate but needs more time and more expensive laboratory equipment than ELISA based kits. In addition, DNA-based techniques do not detect the allergen molecules themselves so do not access the real allergen concentration in the samples.

Evaluations performed over time by different researchers or laboratory analyzes showed that these kits, sometime require improvements. For example, in 1999 Keck-Gassenmeier et al., using a commercially available ELISA kit, showed that with the extraction buffer supplied by the kit only 2-3% of peanut protein added to dark chocolate could be recovered. By addition of fish gelatine into extraction buffer, they obtained recoveries of 60-90% and a detection limit of 2 ppm in dark chocolate improving the test. Similar results were obtained for a wide range of raw materials and finished products [10]. So, for each test kit have to be established the most efficient extraction buffer and to choose the appropriate kit for the samples to be analysed.

An inter-laboratory study was carried out by 31 laboratories in 14 European countries (Austria, Belgium, Switzerland, Czech Republic, Germany, Spain, France, Finland, Greece, Hungary, Norway, Netherlands, Sweden, United Kingdom) using five commercially available peanut ELISA test kits available over the study period. The five test kits have been evaluated by determination and quantification of peanut residues in two food matrices (biscuit and dark chocolate) at different concentrations. Generally, all five ELISA test kits performed well in the concentration range of 5-10 ppm rather than in the low concentration range presented by the manufacturers as LOQ (1-3.3 ppm). The quantification characteristics between test kits differed also significantly at the very low ppm level. Two test kits performed well even at concentrations below 5 ppm with reproducibility of 27-36% for biscuits and 45-57% for chocolate. At three of the five kits some false negative results have been recorded at low concentrations and quantification values beyond the manufacturers' defined cut-off limits. Recoveries of peanut for the different test kits had a spread of 44-191% across all concentrations [11, 12]. It is clear that the type of matrix has a great effect on the capacity of detection/quantification of kits and it is necessary that every kit has to be evaluated by each laboratory before being used in serial analysis. Four of the five ELISA test kits used in inter-laboratory study described above were used to evaluate them in four different matrices: breakfast cereal, milk chocolate, ice cream and cookies. The results obtained were similar with those recorded by the inter-validation study. Two kits were the most accurate and precise kits when results averaged across all protein levels and all food matrixes. It is possible that the differences between data claimed by the manufacturers and those really obtained may appear due to the fact that ten years ago (the period when evaluations were performed) no peanut protein reference standards were commercially available for kits and each manufacturer had to supply a reference standard [13]. A recent study assessed six commercial peanut ELISA kits in order to establish their capacity to recover peanut from a standard reference material (peanut butter) and to detect four major peanut allergens, Ara h 1, Ara h 2, Ara h 3, and Ara h 6. The highest recovery was determined for two kits while the other four shown an underestimate protein content in samples. The kits used shown different sensitivities for the four allergens. Thus, five of the kits were sensitive to Ara h 3 and Ara h 1, while hardly recognizing Ara h 2 and Ara h 6. The sixth kit was sensitive to Ara h 2 and Ara h 6, while showed a very low sensibility to Ara h 1 and Ara h 3 [14]. ELISA kit was also used in different research study, for example to evaluate the peanut allergens in processed food, especially Ara h 1 an Ara h 2. The results showed that, although heat treated peanuts kept part of the allergenic capacity, the commercial ELISA kit used was not able to determine accurately the amount of allergens, mainly because the change in solubility of the target proteins [15-18].

As a general conclusion it can be said that every ELISA test kit has different strengths and limitations and it must be selected the kit that best suits the situational need. In fact, polyclonal ELISA tests are useful tools for screening for peanut but, these are some limitations which arose mainly because the results cannot be directly compared between peanut tests produced by different manufacturers. The solution is the production of international defined allergen standards to be used by all manufacturers.

It has to be specified that Elisa systems are not used only like test kits produced by different manufacturers, on the contrary, scientists often use Enzyme Linked Immunosorbents Assay method preparing themselves different kind of ELISA systems. For example, Pomés A. and her colleagues used a specific 2-site monoclonal antibody for Ara h 1 to develop a sandwich ELISA system. The specific monoclonal antibody-based ELISA realized was used in parallel with a commercial polyclonal ELISA test kit to monitor the Ara h 1 content in food products. The results showed good correlation between the two systems. Because the polyclonal ELISA detected multiple components of peanut, then the most values were well above the standard curve based ELISA and had low sensitivity for Ara h 1. In the meantime monoclonal antibody based ELISA had a sensitivity of 30 ng/ml to 0.34 ng/ml but it is limited only to detect Ara h 1 [19, 20].

A new direction based on ELISA principle is geared to electrochemical immunosensors which are considered as powerful alternatives to ELISA methods for the detection and quantification of allergens although their application in this field is still scarce. For peanut allergens it can be mentioned the electrochemical impedance biosensor for detection of peanut protein Ara h 1 achieved by Huang and his team in 2008. By fitting the impedance spectra to a Randles equivalent circuit, it was demonstrated that the charge transfer resistance (Rct) increases and the differential capacitance (Cd) decreases with increasing concentration of Ara h 1. The detection limit of this reagent less biosensor was estimated to be less than 0.3 nM [21].

Electrochemical immunosensors for Ara h 1 and Ara h 6 were recently developed. Gold nanoparticle-modified screen-printed carbon electrodes were used to develop sandwich-type immunoassay using two-monoclonal antibodies for each allergens Ara h 1 and Ara h 6. The antibody-antigen interaction was detected through the electrochemical detection of enzymatically deposited silver. The limit of detection was of 3.8 for Ara h 1 and 0.27 ng/ml for Ara h 6. The limit of quantification was of 12.6 ng/ml and 0.88 ng/ml for Ara h 1 respectively Ara h 6. In addition, accurate results with recovery of >96.6% for Ara h 1 respectively ≥96.7% for Ara h 6 in complex food matrices (cookies and chocolate) where achieved. The developed biosensors appears as innovative, sensitive, selective, environmentally friendly, cheaper and fast techniques (especially when automated and/or miniaturized), able to effectively replace the classical methodologies [22-24].

Another very new realization is a magnetoimmunosensor based on a sandwich configuration using captured antibodies against Ara h 1, immobilized onto carboxylic acid-modified MBs (HOOC-MBs), and biotinylated detector antibodies. This immunosensor allows a LOD of 6.3 ng/ml and has demonstrated successful applicability for Ara h 1 determination in complex matrices such as diluted food extracts and undiluted saliva samples.

Also, this immunosensor is remarkably faster compared to available commercial ELISA kits, it is flexible, simply and could be mass-produced [25].

The PCR methods and recombining allergens have been used successfully not only to detect peanut allergens in food but also for research, for identification, characterization of old or new allergens. The temporal and spatial regulation mechanism of *Ara h 3* during seed development and genomic structure of this allergen was studied using mainly reverse transcriptase-polymerase chain reaction (RT-PCR) and real-time PCR [26].

The development of genomics and proteomics allows the application of the molecular biology and recombinant DNA in sequencing, synthesis and cloning protein allergens to obtain recombinant allergens. These recombinant allergens play a very important role in discovery, biochemical and structural characterization and assessment of allergic capacity of the new protein identified as allergen. Through this new technology, the epitopes of Ara h 3 were established and well characterized Ara h 5 too [27, 28].

However, at least one of the basically methods like electrophoresis or chromatography techniques is used in almost all research studies for separation, identification and even quantification.

ELECTROMIGRATION METHODS

Proteins analysis requires separation and, for some methods, fractionation processes. The first and the most used separation technique in proteomics is two-dimensional gel electrophoresis followed by chromatography techniques.

Electrophoresis has a long history, with references from 1800s and nowadays it attained the rank of an essential tool for research especially in life sciences domain. Arne Tiselius presented the first sophisticate electrophoresis apparatus and paper about electrophoresis in 1937. He was the first who showed, clearly and unmistakably, the main components of human blood. He received the Nobel Prize in Chemistry for these realisations in 1948. This technique became widely developed in the 1940s and 1950s being used to separate the largest proteins to amino acids and inorganic ions. In 1950 Olivier Smithies invented Gel Electrophoresis and after that a vast amount of ingenious experimental work has been carried out in electrophoresis field with remarkable results and different techniques were developed: SDS-PAGE, Two-dimensional PAGE (2D-PAGE), Isoelectrofocusing (IEF), Fused Rocket Immunoelectrophoresis (FRIE), Crossed Immunoelectrophoresis (CIE), Crossed Radio-Immunoelectrophoresis (CRIE), Capillary Electrophoresis (CE),

Capillary Zone Electrophoresis immunoaffinity capillary electrophoresis (IACE), etc. [29-31]. In consequence electrophoresis studies became a usual method for every research regarding proteins and electrophoresis studies on proteins illustrate the vast amount of research activity in these fields. Gel electrophoresis is usually accomplished for analytical purposes, but it might be used as a preparative technique to partially purify molecules prior to use of other methods such as, PCR, immunoblotting, mass spectrometry or for further characterization.

In this context almost every study regarding allergens has at least a part using electrophoresis methods. Allergen electrophoresis is used to separate, identify, analyse, characterize, and quantify the protein allergens from different sources.

The total protein in samples is evaluated by different methods such as Lowry, Bradford, Kjeldahl, Dumas or Bicinchoninic Acid but these results are rarely presented in papers.

Gel Electrophoresis

In the classical approach gel electrophoresis is a group of techniques used to separate molecules based on physical characteristics such as size, shape, or isoelectric point. In general protein separation is made in two steps. The first step is Isoelectric focusing (IEF) when under the influence of an electrical field charged molecules migrates with different speeds according with charges and masses in the direction of the electrode bearing the opposite charge. The second dimension separation is usually performed by SDS-PAGE which separates according to molecular weight. IEF followed by SDS-PAGE is named two-dimensional electrophoresis (2-DE). This technique was established by O'Farrell in 1975 and represents the core of proteomics technology [32].

This technique can reproducibly separate mixtures of proteins and it is widely used in the first steps to separate, detect, identify and molecular mass establishing for almost all allergens. There are relatively few studies which use only electrophoresis methods for allergens analysis.

So an interesting study regarding the food allergens with low molecular weight presents a simple SDS-PAGE procedure applying it to identify low-molecular weight food-proteins. For example, seven fractions obtained from crude peanut extracts purified by FPLC were analysed using this method. The molecular weight distribution was ranged between 2-17 kDa and for fractions from peanut extracts. The results obtained in 20 replicates by this method were highly reproducible [33].

Various reports have appeared on the purification and identification of peanut allergens. It is known that many food allergens and peanut proteins in particular, are resistant to heat, acidic conditions and gastric digestion. As a result the assessments of food allergens often include the study resistance of the respective allergen to heat, strong acidic conditions and proteases.

Kopper and collaborators studied the resistance of peanut allergens to heat and simulated gastric fluid, pepsin, chymotrypsin and trypsin. Ara h 1 purified by ammonium sulfate precipitation and cation exchange column chromatography, raw peanut and roasted peanut extracts was used. Digested samples were analysed and compared by SDS-PAGE and visualized with Coomassie brilliant blue staining.

Progressive roasting of peanuts resulted in a significant decrease in protein solubility and the digestive tract proteases did not solve it. SDS-PAGE showed that digested Ara h 1 and a crude peanut protein extract, with pepsin and porcine gastric fluid, resulted in the production of nearly identical sets of digestion products by both enzyme sources [34, 35].

To better understand the biochemical and immunochemical characteristics of physiologically occurring forms of Ara h 1, a major allergen from peanut, his structure has to be very well known. In this aim, this allergen was studied a lot regarding his epitopes. It is essential that at least the major allergenic epitopes to be present in protein isolates that are used for the calibration of immunochemical assays, to be sure that no epitopes go undetected in such assays. In this context studies under various extraction and purification conditions were made. In one of these studies Ara h 1 was purified from peanut extract by Gel Permeation Chromatography and Affinity Chromatography and then Ara h 1 was detected by analyzing the fractions with SDS-PAGE using for staining Coomassie Brilliant Blue R 250. After western blotting N-Terminal amino acid sequences were determined. The results obtained permitted to compare the cleaved-off peptide from Ara h 1 with a peptide, designated hypogin, which has antifungal activity and has a substantial homology with the Ara h 1 cleaved-off peptide. Thus it seems that this truncated peptide from Ara h 1 is possibly to be present in peanuts, as an antifungal compound [36].

The resistance of Ara h 1 and Ara h 2 allergens from various peanuts to roasting, boiling and frying was also analyzed comparing the apparent amounts of allergens by SDS-PAGE analysis and the quantities were determined by different quantitative protein content determination methods [37-40].

This situation is determined by some weaknesses of gel electrophoresis regarding proteins analysis such as:

- Electrophoresis conditions generally permit to separate only proteins having molecular masses of 10 kDa and higher;
- It is very difficult (practically impossible) to identify the whole proteome;
- Large, hydrophobic, acidic and basic proteins have difficulties in the movement through the gel and are poor resolved too;
- The highly basic or acidic proteins can abnormal bind to SDS leading to "false" results;
- Proteins existing in the small concentration in sample are usually below the limit of detection of this technique;
- The quantification is still a problem due to the low dynamic range of stains;
- It is not sufficiently accurate and can result in a overestimation or an underestimation of a molecular weight.

These traditional electrophoretic methods are more and more succeeded by capillary electrophoresis.

Capillary Electrophoresis (CE)

Since the technique of capillary electrophoresis was set up CE has become one of the most important methods for detection, quantification and characterisation of proteins/allergens in the last years. The majority of commercial capillary electrophoresis instruments use UV or UV-VIS absorbance for detection but there are more sensitive detection systems as fluorescence, mass spectrometry or Surface-Enhanced Raman Spectroscopy.

Capillary electrophoresis consists of a family of techniques which utilize narrow-bore (20-200 μm i.d.) capillaries and with different considerably operative and separation characteristics to perform high efficiency separations of both large and small molecules. These techniques are: isoelectric focusing, capillary gel electrophoresis, capillary zone electrophoresis, isotachophoresis and micellar electrokinetic capillary chromatography.

In the last years CE coupled with laser-induced fluorescence detection systems for the analysis of proteins has an intense development. Even though the UV absorbance is still used, new alternative methods, like LIF, are tested because of the necessity to find a system which can detect quantities below picomole range. A review regarding this kind of detection which covers the articles published up to 2006 show the instrumentation, laser light sources and the modalities used for nonfluorescent protein and peptide derivatization.

Several proteins and peptides were quantified by these methods but regarding protein allergens it seems that this kind of detection was used only to quantify milk protein allergens, conalbumin and chicken egg albumin. It was shown that using a GaAl/Ar laser diode (785 nm) and near infrared amine labelling reagent the protein could be quantified in range of amol [53].

Some reviews covering many years regarding CE-based techniques coupled with absorption, LIF, and MS detection systems for the analysis of proteins were published. In this review the advantages and disadvantages for protein analysis of each CE technique are emphasized [54, 55].

CE is superior to the other electrophoresis techniques in the separation efficiency, simplicity, low cost of analysis, small amounts of samples required for analysis (a few picograms) and could be completely automated. It is especially useful for separation of peptides and proteins. However, for peanut proteins/allergens, published studies using CE techniques are almost missing.

LIQUID CHROMATOGRAPHY

In the perspective on proteomics and the advances in protein separation techniques, capillary electrophoresis and chromatography (high-performance liquid chromatography, revered-phase chromatography, affinity, ion-exchange chromatography) play an important role. It seems that capillary electrophoresis and HPLC methods will extend faster than other separation methods. Physico-chemical properties of allergens decide the chromatographic procedure which has to be followed to accomplish the best analysis. A review of separation techniques for identification and characterization of allergens evaluated the analytical parameters and emphasized their significance on efficiency of applied procedure [56].

High-performance liquid chromatography (HPLC) could be a proper method for molecular mass determination of allergens size-exclusion. Different kind of chromatography methods to quantify the proteins may perhaps be used but we found that chromatography methods used for quantity determination of allergens/proteins are present only in a few articles.

Size-Exclusion High-Performance Liquid Chromatography and Ion Exchange High-Performance Liquid Chromatography were used mainly for detection and analysis of allergens and not for quantitative determination of it [57].

Recombinant allergens are often produced with aim to use them for *in vivo* and *in vitro* investigations. For quality control, characterization and comparison of recombinant allergen with the native one belong electrophoresis method are used chromatographic methods. Size exclusion chromatography is one of these choices. For example Sec was used to evaluate the products resulted after digestion of Ara h 1 with pepsin at a pH value of 2 [58].

Different kind of High Performance Liquid Chromatography (HPLC), enzyme linked immunoaffinity chromatography (ELIAC) or Immobilized Metal Ion Affinity Chromatography (IMAC) is mainly used for isolation, identification, analysis of composition, extraction and purification of allergens. Using proper condition the quantitative analysis of allergens can be possible by LC techniques. In this chromatographic method retention time is in fact a parameter of chemical structure dependent and is constant in the same working conditions. However these techniques were used mostly for milk, cheese or eggs allergens assessment [59-63].

CIRCULAR DICHROISM

Circular Dichroism (CD) – it is commonly used type of absorption spectroscopy because it is particularly sensitive to configuration and conformation and can be applied to molecules in solution.

Most of researchers use CD especially to characterise the second structure of protein/allergens, their similarities, cross-reactivity, potential hypo-allergenic derivatives, stability of proteins, mutations effects on secondary structure and studies of allergen receptor interactions (antibody-antigen) not to detect them, in different conditions [64-67].

The behaviour of Ara h 1 under gastric conditions was examined in the same study by different methods: SDS-PAGE, SEC and circular dichroism (CD). It was found that peptide fragments (<2 kDa) which survived to proteolytic digestion in acidic medium, formed in basic environment small intestine aggregates which protects and makes epitopes available to triggering an allergic response [58].

Sen and colleagues investigated the secondary and tertiary structural differences between native and reduced Ara h 2 proteins by Circular Dichroism spectra (190-320 nm) at 37°C to see if its disulfide bonds contribute to the secondary and tertiary structure of this protein. The Ara h 2 peanut allergen which was recognized by more than 90% of peanut-allergic patients it has been shown to be resistant to acidic conditions and digestion and its epitopes 3, 6, and 7 were recognized by the majority of peanut allergic people. The data estimates of Sen and colab. showed that secondary structure proportions are 18.2% of the molecule in α-helices, 54% in β-pleated sheet, and 27.7% in a random coil configuration for native Ara h 2 and 82.3% β-pleated sheet and the rest is mostly in a random coil configuration for hydrolyzed Ara h 2. This suggests a dramatically different tertiary structure. However, the Ara h 2 structure is not completely randomized when the disulfide bonds are reduced which means that Ara h 2 is a very ordered protein. Nevertheless the hydrolyzed Ara h 2 lost almost the whole allergenicity [68]. Other authors estimates that the secondary structure for native Ara h 2 is 33% alpha and 3% beta by CD [69] and the allergenicity increases after roasting.

In the meantime a study about conformational changes of Ara h 1 during heat treatment using CD (185-260) showed a completely denaturation of protein similar with a secondary more structured conformation. But heat treatment doesn't affect the allergenicity of Ara h 1 [70]. In a similar way Lehmann and collaborators studied thermal and proteolytic secondary structures changing in the presence of different reagents by CD of Ara h 2 and Ara h 6. They used NMR to analysis the first three structures of these allergens too [71].

In order to improve the diagnoses of allergy and to better understand the properties of allergens researchers often use recombinant allergens. Almost in all cases the second structure of normal and recombinant allergens are studied by CD.

For example, in a previous research, Lehmann and collaborators studied and compared the structure of nAra h 2 to those of rAra h 2 obtained using a special *E. coli BL 21* strain [72].

For the characterization of natural Ara h 8 (nAra h 8) from roasted and unroasted peanuts, circular dichroism spectroscopy, hydrophobic binding assay, immunohistochemistry, and immunoblot with sera of peanut allergic patients were performed and compared with results from recombinant Ara h 8 (rAra h 8) and Bet v 1 [73].

A characterisation of Ara h 9 was done by comparison with similar allergen of peach Pru p 3 using recombinant Arah9 and techniques of electrophoresis, N-terminal amino acid sequencing and circular dichroism spectrometry. CD spectroscopy revealed similar secondary structures of all Ara h 9 isoforms to Pru p 3 [74].

The CD was used to investigate the thermal, saccharides and ions effect on secondary structure of allergens too. Thus CD (200-300 nm) was used to assess the conformational changes of PNA (peanut agglutinin) as a function of low temperatures, saccharides and some ions [75].

Rodriguez-Maranon and collaborators used Magnetic Circular Dichroism to compare the electronic structure of peanut peroxidase (PeP) to horseradish peroxidase isoenzyme C. They found a striking similarity of secondary-structure in the distribution of the predicted helices of the peroxidases even if their primary structure is less than 50% similar [76].

MASS SPECTROMETRY

Nowadays the majority methods used for detection protein allergens imply spectroscopic methods which are highly sensitive and rapid. Currently mass spectrometry is used after identification of allergens by electrophoresis separation immunoblotting and/or chromatography purification to analyse and confirm the identity, molecular mass, post-translational modification characterisation and quantification of allergens found.

The basic scheme of allergens analysis by MS is to separate target allergen/protein by electrophoresis and/or chromatography then significant protein are digested by proteolysis and peptide mixture obtained is analysed by MS for peptide mass fingerprint, peptide sequence, post-translational modification characterisation and quantification. In fact it seems that MS is effectively unique in determining post-translational modifications of food proteins [77].

Mass spectrometry, combined with Liquid chromatography, Matrix-assisted laser desorption/ionization, time-of-flight mass spectrometer or other techniques have been applied to characterize a lot of food proteins and peptides. These techniques can provide molecular mass either of intact proteins or their tryptic peptides. In general modifications (phosphorylation, sulphating, glycosylation, methylation, including multiple formylation provoked by formic acid, cysteine alkylation caused by un-polymerised acrylamide monomers, and complexation with the staining reagents, etc.) are suffered especially by proteins with molecular mass less than 30 kDa [78-82].

The combination of SDS-PAGE with mass spectrometry seems to be a powerful tool for separation, identification, and characterization of proteins. The sensitivity of MS allows protein quantification in the femtomole to attomole range. The great potential of this combination represents a promise for progress in allergen researches [83, 84]. The identification of peanut defensins (Ara h h 12 and Ara h 13) was achieved as well by SDS-PAGE, Western blotting, 2-dimensional PAGE, protein sequencing and mass spectrometry [85].

The identification of proteins by tandem mass spectrometry is developing into database expansion which will allow reducing the number of false negative and false positive identifications [86].

The most legume seeds have as major seed storage proteins vicilins. These proteins have molecular weight from 40 to 70 kd and are usually glycosylated and associated in vivo, forming trimers of 150 to 190 kd. Different posttranslational processing as proteolysis and glycosylation leads to a wide variation in the subunit composition of the oligomers. Similarities between vicillins from different species bring to mind a presumed role of this protein family as plant pan allergens. However it seems that a very clear connection between sequence identity and clinical cross-reactivity was not still established.

One of the most dangerous allergen Ara h 1 is a glycoprotein as the Ole e 1. The analysis of glycoprotein part of these allergens has been reported enough. A study regarding the peptide and glycan mapping of these allergens was achieved by MALDI-MS after tryptic digestion of SDS-PAGE interest bands. Such glycoproteins with N-Glycan structure known horseradish peroxidase (type VI-A), bovine fetuin, bovine ribonuclease B, soybean lectin, leukophytohem-agglutinin and olive pollen were used. The proposed MS method allowed determination of the N-Glycans of Ara h 1 and Ole e 1 and highlighting that both allergens contain only one glycosylation site and while the N-glycans of Ole e 1 are involved in allergenicity those of Ara h 1 aren't [87]. These properties of Ara h 1 and Ole e 1 were illustrated in a study to characterize some glycoproteins SDS-PAGE, MALDI-TOF MS, NMR, HPAEC-PAD and RAST inhibition [88].

In digestive tract proteins, so that and peanut proteins, are broken in peptides by enzymatic digestion. Most of these peptides keep the allergenic activity. In aim to detect the specific peptides biomarkers for peanut protein a liquid chromatography/tandem mass spectrometry (LC/MS/MS) method was developed.

Ara h 1 in a food matrix (Ice Cream) was extracted, protein cleaned up and digested with trypsin. The peptide mixtures obtained were separated on the HPLC column and detected by MS. Mass cut-off filters were used to easily identify and enrich of Ara h 1 in Ice Cream samples. The four most abundant peptides having the following mass/charge ratios, m/z 629.8, m/z 571.3, m/z 606.6, and m/z 869.9 were chosen as biomarkers for Ara h 1. These peptides were chosen because their corresponding sequences were found to be unique to

Ara h 1 and were not identified in any other known protein sequence and had the best intensity and reproducibility of retention time in successive HPLC/MS runs. All of the peptides were detected with a high degree of confidence at the 10 ppm level concentration. So the proposed method could be used for confirmatory test for allergen test kits [89]. Using a similar method peanut allergen Ara h 1 was identified and quantified in dark chocolate by Liquid Chromatography-Tandem Mass Spectrometry too. Improving the detection limit and using single peptide marker concentrations (m/z 688.9) as low as 2 ppm of total protein were detected [90].

To establish the effector activity of Ara h 2, Ara h 6 and their variants, these allergens were extracted by two dimensional gel-electrophoresis and gel filtration methods and then analysed by MALDI-TOF spectrometry [91].

The carbohydrate moieties of glycoproteins can be a cross-reaction source. The structure and molecular mass of N-glycans from 26 plant foods (sweet almonds, apple, asparagus, avocado, banana, buckwheat, carrot, cauliflower, celery, coconut, hazelnut, kiwi, mung bean, onion, orange, papaya, pea, peanut, pear, pine nut, pistachio, potato, soy, strawberry, tomato, walnut) and 1 mushroom were analyse evaluate by MALDI-TOF MS, HPLC and NMR spectroscopy [92].

Matrix assisted laser desorption/ionization–time-of-flight (MALDI–TOF) technique was used to analyse the purified Arachis hypogaea stem lectin (SL-I) and its tryptic digests. It were reported six different isoforms of peanut stem-lectin with very close molecular masses and different pI (4.95, 5.05, 5.20, 5.32, 5.40, 5.92) [93].

It seems that a way to prevent the allergic reactions is immunotherapy by a specific vaccination. To accomplish this, allergen molecules have to be modified either by disrupt allergen structure or by mutation in epitope points. Some fruit allergens were analysed in this way using beside immunochemical methods and SDS-PAGE mass spectrometry.

MS has become popular for biomarker analysis for a number of reasons, including sensitivity and accurate molecular mass determination. Finally, MS has the ability to detect any differences in the sequences of the peptides for potential changes in the immunological response of the food allergen. However, it could be specified that mass spectrometry data alone are not enough for a quantification of individual components.

NUCLEAR MAGNETIC RESONANCE

Nuclear Magnetic Resonance (NMR) is used especially to establish/confirm the structure of the allergens [94, 65], to determine the structure similarities between different allergens, toxins and substances involved in host defences' [95] and the responsibility of structure for cross-reactivity of different plant allergens [96]. The NMR together with gel electrophoresis, N-terminal sequencing, Circular dichroism spectroscopy are used to establish the structure and the stability of Ara h 2 and Ara h 6 [71]. In one experiment which aimed to assess the IgE-binding activity of Peanut lectin (PNA), several types of measurements were used, namely immunoblotting, surface plasmon resonance spectroscopy and ELISA. Some epitopes on the molecular surface of Ara h agglutinin have been identified, epitopes which were recognized by the IgE-containing sera of peanut allergic patients, so these could cause allergic character of PNA. But more studies should be performed to determine with certainty this property [97].

X-RAY CRYSTALLOGRAPHY

The using of a purification technique by crystallization and then X-ray analysis is another way to describe the structure of allergens. However the crystallisation process for one allergen from a complex mixture is a long process that lasts more than 2 weeks [98]. For example X-ray scattering was used to evaluate three versions of Ara h 1 (nAra h 1, rAra h 1 and rsAra h 1) in order to structural characterization of Ara h 1 [99]. X-crystallography is used to establish the allergens structures and epitope predictions together with the Nuclear magnetic Resonance [100]. In fact, X-ray crystallography was used to determine the structure and other allergens in peanuts.

SCANNING ELECTRON MICROSCOPY

Scanning Electron Microscopy is used to analysis and comparison of the microstructure of plan proteins and obviously of allergens [101, 102].

CONCLUSION

The possibility to determine the protein allergen content by other methods than immunochemical or molecular methods appear in fact in a very few articles compared to ELISA or PCR methods.

Due to the widespread presence of protein allergens in food products and the lack of therapies, this threat to sensitive people health represents not only a restriction for quality of life but it is also considered as a severe and challenging problem for the industry with regard to food safety.

In this context in last years a profound interests was showed to initiate a comprehensive set of laws which can control the presence of allergens in food at global level and to ensure that the most potential allergenic ingredients are labelled.

Once isolated and identified as allergen, the protein chemical and biochemical characterization is very often limited mainly by the amount of material available. The necessity to quantify traces of allergen protein in different food resides in the low thresholds which can be dangerous for sensitive people.

After allergenic proteins were identified it is only a problem of time to develop an immunological or molecular method to quantify it in various matrixes. It seems that is the easier way for allergen protein quantification. An alternative method which could be applied at least for a group of similar protein allergens doesn't exist until now. The most common alternative methods found in literature are used as confirmatory methods to immunochemical or molecular methods.

Because these data were often obtained by means of different protocols, the estimation of a real quantity was very difficult. To compare the results of some studies to other of a specific allergen in a complex matrix is difficult the sense that there is only a single independent reference method. Actually the only existent standardised alternative method is the one for milk allergen [103]. This method is based on electrophoresis separation followed by quantification made by visual estimation or better by densitometry.

This review shows that most of alternative methods used to quantify various types of peanut allergens are based on electrophoresis (23.7%), capillary electrophoresis (21.1%), liquid chromatography (34.2%), circular Dichroism (2.6%) and mass spectrometry (18.4%). It should be emphasized that mass spectrometry always was in tandem with other method such as electrophoresis and/or chromatography and was able to quantify extremely low quantities as femtomole or attomole in complex matrixes.

Almost all studies use electrophoresis to characterize allergens and some of them quantify allergens especially by densitometry comparing absorbance intensity of interested spots. The quantitative values are reported as percentage of total protein presented on electropherogram.

A big progress concerning protein quantification is accomplished by capillary electrophoresis. A very low quantity of protein allergens was attended by the capillary electrophoresis with LIF detection systems. This method is extremely promising because it does not only quantify very small traces but it only needs a few minutes to reach that.

More than 30% of alternative methods to quantify protein allergens are based on chromatography, especially on perfusion Reversed Phase High Performance Liquid Chromatography method. The best results obtained by chromatography were those attained using a sandwich enzyme linked immunoaffinity chromatography (ELIAC) by which the amounts of protein detected were in picomole to nanomole level.

The only method we found as regards to protein quantification by Circular Dichroism is a very interesting one because it is a rapid and easy method for detecting allergens and may be possibly used by manufacturers having the advantage that there is no need for critical substances like radioactive isotopes or fluorochromes. In addition with a specific ion and monitoring of ΔCD each protein allergen could be evaluated in a common laboratory.

Methods as liquid chromatography/tandem mass spectrometry (LC/MS/MS) and Q-TOF-MSMS made it possible to detect low levels of allergens up to picomoles and femtomoles in complex matrices as ice cream or fruits. Besides mass spectrometry, it is possible to detect protein allergens after posttranslational modifications.

Nowadays we are still far to have an ideal universal method to detect and quantify the protein traces such as allergens in different matrices but the development of CE coupled with LIF and mass spectrometry is a real promising for the future.

A promising perspective appears in the recent research concerning the allergens electrochemical sensors realisation.

Taking into account that proteomics seems to be one of main area of the future life sciences, the development of alternative methods to quantify and characterize allergens become a part of future strategies.

The success of this domain will also depend strongly on the ability to design and use of new analytical and bioinformatics strategies, which will enable to study in a fast, efficient and accurate manner the huge amount of knowledge about allergens in particular and proteins in general.

REFERENCES

[1]   Allen, K.J., Turner, P.J., Pawankar, R., Taylor, S., Sicherer, S., Lack, G., Rosario, N., Ebisawa, M., Wong, G., Mills, E.N.C., Beyer, K., Fiocchi, A., Sampson, H.A., (2014). Precautionary labelling of foods for allergen content: are we ready for a global framework?. *World Allergy Organ J*, 7:10.

[2]   Steinhart, H., Wigotzki, M., Zunker, K., (2001). Introducing allergists to food chemistry. *Allergy*, 56, Suppl. 67: 9-11.

[3]   Ticha, M., V. Pacakova, Stulik, K., (2002). Proteomics of allergens. *J Chromatogr B Analyt Technol Biomed Life Sci.* 771(1-2): 343-353.

[4]   Poms, R., Anklam, E., (2004). Trends in Detecting Food Allergens. *G.I.T. Laboratory Journal*, 1, 43-46.

[5]   Poms, R. E., Anklam, E., Kuhn, M., (2004). Polymerase chain reaction techniques for food allergen detection. *J AOAC Int.* 87(6), 1391-1397.

[6]   Poms, R.E., Klein, C.L., Anklam, E., (2004). Methods for allergen analysis in food: a review. *Food Addit Contam.* 21(1), 1-31.

[7]   Poms, R.E., Emons, H. Anklam, E., (2006). Reference materials and method validation in allergen detection. Detecting allergens in food. S. J. Koppelman and S. L. Hefle. Cambridge, Woodhead Publishing Limited, 348-356.

[8]   Holzhauser, T., Dehne, L.I., Hoffmann, A., Haustein, D., Vieths, S., (1998). Rocket immunoelectrophoresis (RIE) for determination of potentially allergenic peanut proteins in processed foods as a simple means for quality assurance and food safety. *Zeitschrift für Lebensmitteluntersuchung und - Forschung A*, 206 (1), 1-8.

[9]   Carr, A.C., Moore, S.D., (2012). Lucia, Alejandro, ed. Robust quantification of polymerase chain reactions using global fitting. *PloS ONE*, 7 (5), e37640.

[10] Keck-Gassenmeier, B., Benet, S., Rosa, C., Hischenhuber, C., (1999). Determination of Peanut Traces in Food by a Commercially-available ELISA Test. *Food and Agricultural Immunology*, 11(3), 243-250.

[11] Poms R.E., Agazzi, M.E., Bau, A., Brohee, M., Capelletti, C., Nørgaard, J.V., Anklam, E., (2005). Inter-laboratory validation study of five commercial ELISA test kits for the determination of peanut proteins in biscuits and dark chocolate. *JRC30278, EUR 21577 EN*, http:// publications.jrc.ec.europa.eu/repository/handle/JRC30278.

[12] Poms R.E., Agazzi, M.E., Bau, A., Brohee, M., Capelletti, C., Nørgaard, J.V., Anklam, E., (2005). Inter-laboratory validation study of five

commercial ELISA test kits for the determination of peanut proteins in biscuits and dark chocolate. *Food Additives and Contaminants*, 22(2), 104-112.

[13] Whitaker, T.B., Williams, K.M., Trucksess, M.W., Slate, A.B., (2005). Immunochemical analytical methods for the determination of peanut proteins in foods. *Journal of AOAC International*, 88(1), 161-174.

[14] Jayasena, S., Smits, M., Fiechter, D., de Jong, A., Nordlee, J., Baumert, J., Taylor, S.L., Pieters, R.H., Koppelman, S.J., (2015). Comparison of Six Commercial ELISA Kits for Their Specificity and Sensitivity in Detecting Different Major Peanut Allergens. *J. Agric. Food Chem.*, 63 (6), 1849-1855.

[15] Fu, T-J., Maks, N., (2013). Impact of thermal processing on ELISA detection of peanut allergens. *J. Agric. Food Chem.*, 61(24), 5649-5658.

[16] Montserrat, M., Mayayo, C., Sánchez, L., Calvo M., Pérez, M.D., (2013). Study of thermoresistance of the allergenic Ara h 1protein from peanut (Arachis hypogaea). *J. Agric. Food Chem.*, 61(13), 3335-3340.

[17] Montserrat, M., Sanz, D., Juan, T., Herrero, A., Sánchez, L., Calvo, M., Pérez M.D., (2015). Detection of peanut (Arachis hypogaea) allergens in processed foods by immunoassay: influence of selected target protein and ELISA format applied. *Food Control*, 54, 300-330.

[18] Schmitt, D.A., Nesbit, J.B., Hurlburt, B.K., Cheng, H., Maleki, S.J., (2010). Processing can alter the properties of peanut extract preparations. *J Agric Food Chem*, 58(2), 1138-1143.

[19] Pomés, A., Helm, R.M., Bannon, G.A., Burks, A.W., Tsay, A., Chapman, M.D. (2003). Monitoring peanut allergen in food products by measuring Ara h 1. *J Allergy Clin Immunol*, 111(3), 640-645.

[20] Peng, J., Song, S., Xu, L., Ma, W., Liu, L., Kuang, H., Xu, C., (2013). Development of a Monoclonal Antibody-Based Sandwich ELISA for Peanut Allergen Ara h 1 in Food. *Int. J. Environ. Res. Public Health*, 10, 2897-2905.

[21] Huang, Y., Bell, M.C., Suni, I.I., (2008). Impedance biosensor for peanut protein Ara h 1. *Anal. Chem.* 80, 9157-9161.

[22] Alves, R.C., Barroso, M.F., González-García, M.B., Oliveira, M.B.P.P., Delerue-Matos, C., (2015). New Trends in Food Allergens Detection: Towards Biosensing Strategies. *Critical Reviews in Food Science and Nutrition*, Online: http://www.tandfonline.com/doi/full/10.1080/10408 398.2013.831026.

[23] Alves, R.C., Pimentel, F.B., Nouws, H.P.A., Correr, W., González-García, M.B., Oliveira, M.B.P.P., Delerue-Matos, C., (2015). Detection

of the peanut allergen Ara h 6 in foodstuffs using a voltammetric biosensing approach. *Anal. Bioanal. Chem*, 407(23), 7157-7163.

[24] Alves, R.C., Pimentel, F.B., Nouws, H.P.A., Marques, R.C.B., González-García, M.B., Oliveira, M.B.P.P., Delerue-Matos, C., (2015). Detection of Ara h 1 (a major peanut allergen) in food using an electrochemical gold nanoparticle-coated screen-printed immunosensor. *Biosens. Bioelectron.* 64, 19-24.

[25] Montiel, V.R.-V., Campuzano, S., Pellicanò, A., Torrente-Rodriguez, R.M., Reviejo, A.J., Cosio, M.S., Pingarrón, J.M., (2015). Sensitive and selective magnetoimmunosensing platform for determination of the food allergen Ara h 1, *Anal. Chim. Acta,* in press, Online: http://dx.doi.org/10. 1016/j.aca.2015.04.041.

[26] Fu, G., Zhong, Y., Li, C., Li, Y., Lin, X., Liao, B., Tsang, E.W.T., Wu, K., Huang, S., (2010). Epigenetic regulation of peanut allergen gene *Ara h 3* in developing embryos. *Planta*, 231, 1049-1060.

[27] Rabjohn, P., Helm, E.M.Stanley, J.S., West, C.M., Sampson, H.A., Burks, A.W., Bannon, G.A., (1999). Molecular cloning and epitope analysis of the peanut allergen Ara h 3. *J. Clin. Invest.,* 103, 535-542.

[28] Cabanos, C., Tandang-Silvas, M. R., Odijk, V., Brostedt, P., Tanaka, A., Utsumi, S., Maruyama, N. (2010). Expression, purification, cross-reactivity and homology modeling of peanut profilin. *Protein Expr Purif*, 73(1), 36-45.

[29] Bier, M., editor (1959). "Electrophoresis, Theory, Methods and Applications." Academic Press NY.

[30] Baczek, T., (2005). Improvement of Peptides Identification in Proteomics with the Use of New Analytical and Bioinformatic strategies. *Curr Pharm Anal.* 1, 31-40.

[31] Gasilova, N., Girault, H.H., (2015). Bioanalytical methods for food allergy diagnosis, allergen detection and new allergen discovery. *Bioanalysis,* 7(9), 1175-1190.

[32] O'Farrell, P.H., (1975). High resolution two-dimensional electrophoresis of proteins. *J Biol Chem.* 250(10), 4007-4021.

[33] Dean, T.P., Clarke, M.C., Hourihane, J.O'B., Dean, K.R., Warner, J.O., (1996). Application of an electrophoretic methodology for the identification of low molecular weight proteins in foods. *Pediatr Allergy Immunol* 7(4), 171-175.

[34] Kopper, R.A., Odum, N.J., Sen, M., Helm, R.M., Stanley, J.S., Burks, W.A., (2004). Peanut protein allergens: gastric digestion is carried out exclusively by pepsin. *J Allergy Clin Immunol.* 114(3), 614-618.

[35] Kopper, R.A., Odum, N.J., Sen, M., Helm, R.M., Stanley, J.S., Burks, A.W. (2005). Peanut protein allergens: the effect of roasting on solubility and allergenicity. *Int Arch Allergy Immunol*, 136(1): 16-22.

[36] Wichers, H.J., de Beijer, T., Savelkoul, H.F.J., van Amerongen, A., (2004). The major peanut allergen Ara h 1 and its cleaved-off N-terminal peptide; possible implications for peanut allergen detection. *J Agric Food Chem*, 52(15), 4903-4907.

[37] Beyer, K., Morrow, E. et al. (2001). Effects of cooking methods on peanut allergenicity. *J Allergy Clin Immunol*. 107(6), 1077-1081.

[38] Chassaigne, H., Brohée, M., Nørgaard, J.V., van Hengel, A.J., (2007). Investigation on sequential extraction of peanut allergens for subsequent analysis by ELISA and 2D gel electrophoresis. *Food Chemistry*, 105, 1671-1681.

[39] Teodorowicz, M., Fiedorowicz, E., Kostyra, H., Wichers, H., Kostyra, E. (2013). Effect of Maillard reaction on biochemical properties of peanut 7S globulin (Ara h 1) and its interaction with a human colon cancer cell line (Caco-2). *Eur J Nutr*. 52, 1927-1938.

[40] Maleki, S.J., Schmitt, D.A., Galeano, M., Hurlburt B.K. (2014). Comparison of the Digestibility of the Major Peanut Allergens in Thermally Processed Peanuts and in Pure Form. *Foods*, 3, 290-303.

[41] Koppelman, S. J., Vlooswijk, R. A. Knippels, M.J., Hessing, M., Knol, E.F., Van Reijsen, F.C., Bruijnzeel-Koomen, C.A.F.M., (2001). Quantification of major peanut allergens Ara h 1 and Ara h 2 in the peanut varieties Runner, Spanish, Virginia, and Valencia, bred in different parts of the world. *Allergy* 56(2), 132-137.

[42] Basha, S., (1992). Effect of Location and Season on Peanut Seed Protein and Polypeptide Composition. *J. Agric. Food Chem*. 40, 1784-1788.

[43] Walczyk, N.E., Smith, P.M.C., Tovey, E., Wright, G.C., Fleischfressee, D.B., Roberts, T.H., (2013). Analysis of crude protein and allergen abundance in peanuts (*Arachis hypogaea* cv. Walter) from three growing regions in Australia. *J. Agric. Food Chem*. 61(15), 3714-3725.

[44] Magni, C., Ballabio, C., Restani, P., Sironi, E., Scarafoni, A., Poiesi, C., Duranti, M., (2005). Two-dimensional electrophoresis and western-blotting analyses with anti Ara h 3 basic subunit IgG evidence the cross-reacting polypeptides of Arachis hypogaea, Glycine max, and Lupinus albus seed proteomes. *J Agric Food Chem*. 53(6), 2275-2281.

[45] Laemmli, U. (1970). Cleavage of structural proteins during the assembly of the head of bacteriophage T4. *Nature*, 227. 680-685.

[46] Suhr, M., D. Wicklein Lepp, U., Becker, W-M., (2004). Isolation and characterization of natural Ara h 6: evidence for a further peanut allergen with putative clinical relevance based on resistance to pepsin digestion and heat. *Mol Nutr Food Res.*, 48(5), 390-399.

[47] Pons, L., Olszewski, A., Guéant, J-L., (1998). Characterization of the oligomeric behavior of a 16.5 kDa peanut oleosin by chromatography and electrophoresis of the iodinated form. *J Chromatogr B Biomed Sci Appl.*, 706(1), 131-140.

[48] Schwager, C., Kull1, S., Krause1, S., Schocker, F., Petersen, A., Becker, W-M., Jappe, U., (2015). Development of a Novel Strategy to Isolate Lipophilic Allergens (Oleosins) from Peanuts. *PLoS ONE*, 10(4):e01234 19.

[49] Lotan, R., Skutelsky, E., Danon, D., Sharon, N., (1975). The purification, composition, and specificity of the anti-T lectin from peanut (*Arachis hypogaea*). *J Biol Chem.*, 250(21), 8518-8523.

[50] Ruebelt, M.C., Leimgruber, N.K., Lipp, M., Reynolds, T.L., Nemeth, M.A., Astwood, J.D., Engel, K-H., Jany, K-D., (2006). Application of two-dimensional gel electrophoresis to interrogate alterations in the proteome of genetically modified crops. 1. Assessing analytical validation. *J Agric Food Chem.* 54(6), 2154-2161.

[51] Ruebelt, M.C., Lipp, M., Reynolds, T.L., Astwood, J.D., Engel, K-H., Jany, K-D., (2006). Application of two-dimensional gel electrophoresis to interrogate alterations in the proteome of genetically modified crops. 2. Assessing natural variability. *J Agric Food Chem.*, 54(6), 2162-2168.

[52] Ruebelt, M.C., Lipp, M., Reynolds, T.L., Schmuke, J.J., Astwood, J.D., DellaPenna, D., Engel, K-H., Jany, K-D., (2006). Application of two-dimensional gel electrophoresis to interrogate alterations in the proteome of gentically modified crops. 3. Assessing unintended effects. *J Agric Food Chem.*, 54(6), 2169-2177.

[53] Garcia-Campana, A. M., Taverna, M., Fabre, H., (2007). LIF detection of peptides and proteins in CE. *Electrophoresis*, 28(1-2), 208-232.

[54] Huang, Y.F., Huang, C.C., Hu, C-C., Chang, H-T., (2006). Capillary electrophoresis-based separation techniques for the analysis of proteins. *Electrophoresis*, 27(18), 3503-3522.

[55] Dolnik, V., (2006). Capillary electrophoresis of proteins 2003-2005. *Electrophoresis*, 27, 126-141.

[56] Pacakova, V., Stulik, K., Tichá, M., (1997). High-performance separations in isolation and characterization of allergens. *J Chromatogr B Biomed Sci Appl.*, 699(1-2), 403-418.

[57] Bassoli, A., Chioccara, F., Di Gregorio, G., Rindone, B., Tollari, S., Falagiani, P., Riva, G., Bolzachini, E., (1988). Analysis of allergenic components of a Parietaria judaica pollen extract by chromatographic methods for the evaluation of purification procedures. *J Chromatogr.*, 444, 209-218.

[58] Khan, I.J., Di, R., Patel, P., Nanda, V., (2013). Evaluating disulfide crosslinking and pH-induced aggregation of *Arachis hypogea* 1 as components of Peanut Allergy. *J Agric Food Chem.*, 61(35), 8430-8435.

[59] Garcia, M.C., Marina, M.L., Torre, M., (1997). Simultaneous separation of soya bean and animal whey proteins by reversed-phase high-performance liquid chromatography. Quantitative analysis in edible samples. *Anal Chem.*, 69(11), 2217-2220.

[60] Garcia, M.C., Marina, M.L., Torre, M., (1998). Ultrarapid detection of bovine whey proteins in powdered soybean milk by perfusion reversed-phase high-performance liquid chromatography. *J Chromatogr A*, 822 (2), 225-232.

[61] Bordin, G., Cordeiro Raposo, F., de la Calle, B., Rodriguez, A.R., (2001). Identification and quantification of major bovine milk proteins by liquid chromatography. *J Chromatogr. A,* 928(1), 63-76.

[62] Prošková, A., Kucera, J., (2002). Immobilized Metal Ion Chromatographic (IMAC) Determination of Ovomucoid in Hen's Egg White. *Czech. J. Food Sci.* 20(3), 95-97.

[63] Puerta, A., Diez-Masa, J.C., de Frutos, M., (2006). Immunochromatographic determination of ß-lactoglobulin and its antigenic peptides in hypoallergenic formulas. *International Dairy Journal*, 16(5), 406-414.

[64] Flicker, S., Vrtala, S., Steinberger, P., Vangelista, L., Bufe, A., Petersen, A., Ghannadan, M., Sperr, W.R., Valent, P., Norderhaug, L., Bohle, B., Stockinger, H., Suphioglu, C., Ong, E.K., Kraft, D., Valenta, R., (2000). A human monoclonal IgE antibody defines a highly allergenic fragment of the major timothy grass pollen allergen, Phl p 5: molecular, immunological, and structural characterization of the epitope-containing domain. *J Immunol.* 165(7), 3849-3859.

[65] Barral, P., Tejera, M.L., Treviño, M.A., Batanero, E., Villalba, M., Bruix, M., Rodriguez, R., (2004). Recombinant expression of Ole e 6, a Cys-enriched pollen allergen, in Pichia pastoris yeast: detection of partial oxidation of methionine by NMR. *Protein Expr Purif.* 37(2), 336-343.

[66] Mittag D, Akkerdaas J, Ballmer-Weber BK, Vogel L, Wensing M, Becker WM, Koppelman, S.J., Knulst, A.C., Helbling, A., Hefle, S.L., van Ree,

R., Vieths, S., (2004). Ara h 8, a Bet v 1-homologous allergen from peanut, is a major allergen in patients with combined birch pollen and peanut allergy. *J Allergy Clin Immunol.* 114(6):1410-1417.

[67] Verdino, P., Keller, W. (2004). Circular dichroism analysis of allergens. *Methods*, 32(3), 241-248.

[68] Sen, M., Kopper, R., Pons, L., Abraham, E.C., Burks, A. W., Bannon, G.A., (2002). Protein structure plays a critical role in peanut allergen stability and may determine immunodominant IgE-binding epitopes. *J Immunol*, 169(2), 882-887.

[69] Maleki, S.J., Hurlburt, B.K., (2004). Structural and functional alterations in major peanut allergens caused by thermal processing. *J AOAC Int.*, 87 (6): 1475-1479.

[70] Koppelman, S.J., Bruijnzeel-Koomen, C.A., Hessing, M., de Jongh, H.H., (1999). Heat-induced conformational changes of Ara h 1, a major peanut allergen, do not affect its allergenic properties. *J Biol Chem*, 274 (8), 4770-4777.

[71] Lehmann, K., Schweimer, K., Reese, G., Randow, S., Suhr, M., Becker, W-M., Vieths, S., Rösch, P., (2006). Structure and stability of 2S albumin-type peanut allergens: implications for the severity of peanut allergic reactions. *Biochem J.*, 395(3), 463-472.

[72] Lehmann, K., Hoffmann, S., Neudecker, P., Suhr, M., Becker, W-M., Rösch, P., (2003). High-yield expression in Escherichia coli, purification, and characterization of properly folded major peanut allergen Ara h 2. *Protein Expr Purif.* 31(2), 250-259.

[73] Petersen, A., Rennert, S., Kull, S., Becker, W. M., Notbohm, H., Goldmann, T., Jappe, U. (2014). Roasting and lipid binding provide allergenic and proteolytic stability to the peanut allergen Ara h 8. *Biol Chem.*, 395(2), 239-250.

[74] Lauer, I., Dueringer, N., Pokoj, S., Rehm, S., Zoccatelli, G., Reese, G., Moncin, M., Bahima, C., Enrique, E., Lidholm, J., Vieths, S., Scheurer, S., (2009). The non-specific lipid transfer protein, Ara h 9, is an important allergen in peanut. *Clin. Exp. Allergy*, 39(9), 1427-1437.

[75] Decastel, M., Bourrillon, R., Frénoy J.P., (1981). Cryoinsolubility of peanut agglutinin. Effect of saccharides and neutral salts. *J Biol Chem.* 256(17), 9003-9008.

[76] Rodriguez-Maranon, M.J., Mercier, D., van Huystee, R.B., Stillman, M.J., (1994). Analysis of the optical absorption and magnetic-circular-dichroism spectra of peanut peroxidase: electronic structure of a

peroxidase with biochemical properties similar to those of horseradish peroxidase. *Biochem J.*, 301(Pt 2), 335-341.

[77] Ferranti, P., (2004). Mass spectrometric approach for the analysis of food proteins. *Eur J Mass Spectrom (Chichester, Eng)*, 10(3), 349-358.

[78] Galvani, M., Bordini, E., Piubelli, C., Hamdan, M., (2000). Effect of experimental conditions on the analysis of sodium dodecyl sulphate polyacrylamide gel electrophoresis separated proteins by matrix-assisted laser desorption/ionisation mass spectrometry. *Rapid Commun Mass Spectrom.* 14(1), 18-25.

[79] Galvani, M., Hamdan M., (2000). Electroelution and passive elution of gamma-globulins from sodium dodecyl sulphate polyacrylamide gel electrophoresis gels for matrix-assisted laser desorption/ionisation time-of-flight mass spectrometry. *Rapid Commun Mass Spectrom.*, 14(8), 721-723.

[80] Galvani, M., Hamdan, M., righetti, P.G., (2000). Two-dimensional gel electrophoresis/matrix-assisted laser desorption/ionisation mass spectrometry of a milk powder. *Rapid Commun Mass Spectrom.*, 14(20), 1889-1897.

[81] Leonil, J., Gagnaire, V., Mollé, D., Pezennec, S., Bouhallab, S., (2000). Application of chromatography and mass spectrometry to the characterization of food proteins and derived peptides. *J Chromatogr A*, 881(1-2), 1-21.

[82] Kuhner, S., Gavin A-C., (2007). Towards quantitative analysis of proteome dynamics. *Nature Biotechnology*, 25(3), 298-300.

[83] Crameri, R., (2005). The potential of proteomics and peptidomics for allergy and asthma research. *Allergy*, 60(10), 1227-1237.

[84] Veenstra, T., (2006). Proteomics for Biological Discovery, eds. Veenstra, T.D. and Yates, J.R., John Wiley and Sons, Inc.

[85] Petersen, A., Kull, S., Rennert, S., Becker, W-M., Susanne Krause, S., Ernst, M., Gutsmann, T., Bauer, J., Lindner, B., Jappe, U., (2015). Peanut defensins: Novel allergens isolated from lipophilic peanut extract. *J Allergy Clin Immunol,* 9 June – in press, http://dx.doi.org/10. 1016/j.jaci.2015.04.010.

[86] Hernandez, P., Muller, M., Appel, R.D., (2006). Automated protein identification by tandem mass spectrometry: issues and strategies *Mass Spectrometry Reviews* 25, 235-254.

[87] Kolarich, D., Altmann, F., (2000). N-Glycan analysis by matrix-assisted laser desorption/ionization mass spectrometry of electrophoretically

separated nonmammalian proteins: application to peanut allergen Ara h 1 and olive pollen allergen Ole e 1. *Anal Biochem*, 285(1), 64-75.

[88] van Ree, R., Cabanes-Macheteau, M., Akkerdaas, J., Milazzo, J-P., Loutelier-Bourhis, C., Rayon, C., Villalba, M., Koppelman, S., Aalberse, R., Rodriguez, R., Faye, L., Lerouge, P., (2000). Beta(1,2)-xylose and alpha(1,3)-fucose residues have a strong contribution in IgE binding to plant glycoallergens. *J Biol Chem.*, 275(15), 11451-11458.

[89] Shefcheck, K.J., Musser, S.M. (2004). Confirmation of the allergenic peanut protein, Ara h 1, in a model food matrix using liquid chromatography/tandem mass spectrometry (LC/MS/MS). *J Agric Food Chem.* 52(10), 2785-2790.

[90] Shefcheck, K.J., Callahan, J.H., Musser, S.M., (2006). Confirmation of peanut protein using peptide markers in dark chocolate using liquid chromatography-tandem mass spectrometry (LC-MS/MS). *J Agric Food Chem.* 54(21), 7953-7999.

[91] Porterfield, H.S., Murray, K.S., Schlichting, D.G., Chen, X., Hansen, K.C., Duncan, M.W., Dreskin, S.C., (2009). Effector activity of peanut allergens: a critical role for Ara h 2, Ara h 6, and their variants. *Clin Exp Allergy*, 39(7), 1099-1108.

[92] Wilson, I.B., Altmann, F. (1998). Structural analysis of N-glycans from allergenic grass, ragweed and tree pollens: core alpha1,3-linked fucose and xylose present in all pollens examined. *Glycoconj J.*, 15(11), 1055-1070.

[93] Agrawal, P., Kumar, S., Das, H.R., (2010). Mass spectrometric characterization of isoform variants of peanut (*Arachis hypogaea*) stem lectin (SL-I). *Journal of Proteomics,* 73(6), 1573-1586.

[94] Faber, C., Lindemann, A. Sticht, H., Ejchart, A., Kungl, A., Susani, M., Frank, R.W., Kraft, D., Breitenbach, M., Rösch, P., (1996). Secondary structure and tertiary fold of the birch pollen allergen Bet v 1 in solution. *J Biol Chem.* 271(32), 19243-19250.

[95] Furmonaviciene, R., Shakib, F., (2001). The molecular basis of allergenicity: comparative analysis of the three dimensional structures of diverse allergens reveals a common structural motif. *Mol Pathol.*, 54(3), 155-159.

[96] Jenkins, J.A., Griffiths-Jones, S., Shewry, P.R., Breitender, H., Mills, C., (2005). Structural relatedness of plant food allergens with specific reference to cross-reactive allergens: an in silico analysis. *J Allergy Clin Immunol.* 115(1), 163-170.

[97] Rouge, P., Culerrier, R., Granier, C., Rance, F., Barre, A., (2010). Characterization of IgE-binding epitopes of peanut (Arachis hypogaea) PNA lectin allergen cross-reacting with other structurally related legume lectins. *Mol Immunol.* 47(14), 2359-2366.

[98] Bufe, A., Betzel, C., Schramm, G., Petersen, A., Becker, W.-M., Schlaak, M., Perbandt, M., Dauter, Z., Weber, W., (1996). Crystallization and preliminary diffraction data of a major pollen allergen. Crystal growth separates a low molecular weight form with elevated biological activity. *J Biol Chem.*, 271(44), 27193-27196.

[99] Chruszcz, M., Maleki, S.J., Majorek, K.A., Demas, M., Bublin, M., Solberg, R., Hurlburt, B.K., Ruan, S., Mattisohn, C.P., Breiteneder, H., Minor, W., (2011). Structural and Immunologic Characterization of Ara h 1, a Major Peanut Allergen. *J. Biol. Chem.*, 286(45), 39318-39327.

[100] Dall'Antonia, F., Pavkov-Keller, T., Zangger, K., Keller, W., (2014). Structure of allergens and structure based epitope predictions. *Methods*, 66, 3-21.

[101] Vrtala, S., Hirtenlehner, K., Susani, M., Mübeccel, A., Kussebi, F., Akdis, C.A., Blaser, K., Hufnagl, P., Binder, B.R., Politou, A., pastore, A., Vangelista, L., Sperr, W.R., Semper, H., Valent, P., Ebner, C., Kraft, D., Valenta, R., (2001). Genetic engineering of a hypoallergenic trimer of the major birch pollen allergen Bet v 1. *Faseb J.*, 15(11), 2045-2047.

[102] Gorinstein S., P. E., Delgado-Licon E., Yamamoto K., Kobayashi S., Taniguchi H., Haruenkit R., Park Y.-S., Jung S-T., Drzewiecki J., Trakhtenberg S., (2004). Use of scanning electron microscopy to indicate the similarities and differences in pseudocereal and cereal proteins. *Int J Food Sci Tech*, 39(2), 183-189.

[103] Regulation, C. (2001). Reference method for the detection of cows' milk and caseinate in cheeses from ewes' milk, goats' milk or buffalos' milk or mixtures of ewes,' goats' and buffalos' milk. *Official Journal of the European Communities*, L037 (no.213): p.P1, Annex XV.

In: Peanut Allergies
Editors: M. Pele and C. Cimpeanu

ISBN: 978-1-63484-742-1
© 2016 Nova Science Publishers, Inc.

Chapter 5

PEANUT ALLERGIES: PREVENTION

*Elena Maria Draghici, PhD**
University of Agronomic Sciences and Veterinary
Medicine Bucharest

ABSTRACT

Avoiding specific foods and ingredients to which patients are allergic poses an important health challenge. The prevalence of peanut allergy is increasing worlewide. This has a significant impact on life quality, as different countries are governed by different manufacturing regulations and guidelines. Peanut allergy is high and there is currently no treatment for it. The lethal risk associated with peanut allergy and in order to protect public health led the regulatory bodies worldwide to issue legislation concerning requirement to clearly warned on label the possible presence of food allergens, therefore those of peanut too. A number of regulations address peanut allergy worldwide and aim to mitigate risk to consumers. In addition, different organisations were created in order to learn and to protect sensitive people.

Keywords: peanuts, legislation, labelling

---

* Corresponding Author address: Email: draghiciem@yahoo.com.

PREVENTION

In general, allergies are caused by a series of substances, however in all the cases they are based on a protein to which the body reacts aggressively. In some cases, the allergen can cause an even deadly anaphylactic shock; the peanut allergies belong to this category.

Regarding the allergen quality, i.e., peanuts, required for triggering the allergic symptoms, it is known that the individuals which are the most sensitive to allergy react to amounts of micrograms, milligrams, or even smaller amounts.

The importance of approaching the food allergies varies depending on the country and the type of food.

Peanuts can cause or induce allergies, especially in children. In the latest years, they have performed studies in order to identity how many children, especially, have food allergies. This is important because the frequency of the allergies occurrence is much higher as compared to approx. 30-40 years ago, and at present, almost every child suffers from one food allergy. The statistical data have proved that, during 1997-2008, the increase rate of the peanut allergy has almost tripled from approx. 0.4% to 1.4%.

Statistics have proved that, during 1997-2008, the increase rate to the peanut allergy has progressively increased, and almost tripled from approx. 0.4% in 1998 to 1.2% in 2002 and to 1.4% in 2008. In the subjects under 18 years old, a higher percentage has been found as compared to the adult population [1].

From the data reported in the USA in 1999 in the Journal of Allergy & Clinical Immunology (JACI), it is estimated that 1% of the population, about 3 million Americans, are allergic to peanuts or nuts. In 2005, they have recorded in the edition Food Allergy News, a publication of FAAN (Food Allergy & Anaphylaxis Network), 11.4 million allergic Americans, i.e., 4% of the world population.

The importance given to this allergy has increased as, during 1997-2002, the number of allergic persons has doubled, according to the statistics reported in December 2003 in JACI. It is presumed that the people's immunity system has decreased at the same time as the development of civilization. The researchers do not really know what has caused this but it is presumed that, because of the peanuts roasting technology, the allergic effect of the peanuts is much stronger as compared to the blanching or boiling treatment used in China.

The most famous peanuts manufacturing countries are: China, Indonesia, Korea, Pakistan, Thailand, Israel, etc.

High percentages of peanut allergy occurrence have been found in all geographical areas, i.e., Asia, Middle East, Africa, South America, but not all the countries in the geographical areas have recorded a high allergy occurrence frequency [2].

The studies performed by several researchers have shown that only in some states they have recorded a high frequency of the peanut allergy exclusively, as compared to the rest of nuciferous trees. They have recorded:

- In Asia, in countries like China [3], Hong Kong, Thailand, Taiwan [4], Malaysia [3], Singapore (1.2%), and the Philippines (5.1%).
- In the Middle East, in Saudi Arabia [5];
- In Africa, Zimbabwe [6], Morocco [7], Ghana [8] in 5% of the children, they have identified the peanut and pineapple allergy [8];
- South Africa [9] and Egypt [10];
- South America – only in Brazil and Mexico they have recorded, besides the other types of allergies, also the peanut allergy [11, 12, 13].

Based on these statistical arguments, in order to protect the population, it has been required to issue normative documents guaranteeing the correct information of the consumer, in order to prevent the possible allergic occurrences.

In 2004, they have adopted the legislation regarding the marking of the allergens by clear labeling, so that a child over 7 years old could understand the content of the ingredients.

Practically, the status of the regulations regarding the peanut allergies, strictly referring to this product, imposes the certainty that the consumer is fully informed.

According to the above, it is clear that we have to grant special attention to allergenicity when assessing the safety of the food.

The Legislation Regarding the Peanut Allergies

Considering the importance of information regarding the risk of this type of allergy, and in order to prevent possible risks, it has become necessary to label the food.

The inspections agreed upon at the EU level regarding the food labeling have been enforced starting with Directive 79/112 in 1979, and additional inspections as well as modifications made have also been added, in order to provide a wide range of labeling requirements. In 2000, CE has adopted

Directive no.13. Additional directives regarding labeling have also been adopted.

The states belonging to the European Economic Area (EEA) have incorporated the EU legislation regulating the labeling of the food products, according to the Agreement regarding the Economic European Area.

The new regulations regarding food labeling are part of a package of no less than 68 normative documents which have been adopted by the EEA countries.

The purpose of these legislative norms is to regulate the food labeling in such a way that consumers would have easier access to information. Before making choices based on a correct documentation when purchasing food, consumers should have essential information available, legible and easy to understand.

Food Labeling According to the EU Legislation

The European Union (EU) has established new food labeling rules, so that all European consumers would be informed on the allergen ingredients when deciding to purchase a certain food product.

The rules are meant to provide comprehensive information on the food products you purchase. Except for the information legally requested, the manufacturers are free to provide any other information they choose, as long as it is accurate, and is not misleading for the consumers. There are labeling rules enforceable to all types of food, as well as particular rules for meat, alcohol and perishable food.

The purpose of labeling is to correctly inform the consumers; the mandatory information which must be included by the label is:

1. Identity + contents + features of the product;
2. Date of minimal validity; Preservation conditions, safety in use; Ingredients which can damage the health of certain categories of consumers; Risks and consequences;
3. Nutritional features.

The information meant for the consumers must be clear, easy to understand, placed in the main visual field, legible, and must include mandatory but also additional information. The height of the letters must be at least 1.2 mm (except for the small packages or containers).

The label must be legible, and must include:

- The name of the product (scientific and commercial in the case of peanuts) must include information on the physical state of the food or particular treatment to which it has been subject to (as powder, frozen, concentrate, etc.). The ionization treatment must always be mentioned, if used.
- The list of ingredients must include all ingredients, and these must be enumerated in the decreasing order of their weight (exception: mixes of fruits and vegetables), including those known to cause reactions in allergic persons (e.g., peanuts, milk, eggs, and fish).
- Amount of ingredients.
- Allergens with a risk of intolerance.
- Net amount per product.
- Consumption deadline (validity).
- The comments "expiry date" and "best preferably before" shows for how long the food stays fresh and under safety conditions for consumption. The comment "expiry date" is used for the food which is deteriorated within a certain period of time. All packed fresh products have the comment "expiry date". You should not eat products after the expiry date, because you might suffer from food poisoning. The comment "Best preferably before" is used for products which can be preserved for a longer time (e.g., cereals, rice, spices, and peanuts). It is not dangerous to eat products after this date, but the products might lose their flavor and structure.
- For the ecological production, one shall definitely use the expression "ecological production". Showing it on labels is strongly regulated by the EU legislation. It is only allowed in relation to specific methods of food production, which fulfill high standards of environmental protection and animal welfare. The European logo "Ecological agriculture – EC control system" can be used by the manufacturers fulfilling the required conditions.
- For the Genetically Modified Organisms (GMOs): the labeling is mandatory for the products having a GMO content of over 0.9%. All the GMO substances must be mentioned in the list of ingredients using the words "genetically modified".

Preservation Conditions

- Nutritional values and specifications regarding the nutritional and health benefits. The energy value and the nutritional elements of the food (e.g., proteins, fat, fibers, sodium, vitamins and minerals) are indicated.
- The name and address of the manufacturer, of the packer or importer must eligibly be mentioned on the package, so that one could know who they could contact in case of a complaint, or for additional information about the product.
- Country or place of origin
- Please indicate the name of the country or of the region of origin. Also, it is mandatory, if the trade name or other elements on the label, such as an image, a flag, or a reference to a certain place, might mislead the consumers about the real origin of the product.

Labeling of Food Products

The European Union (EU) improves its regulations concerning the labeling of food products, so that the consumer may get essential, legible and easy to understand information to be able to purchase products knowing well what he purchases. For reasons of public health, the new regulations consolidate the protection against allergens. The ingredients containing peanuts are the ones that are mainly responsible for the occurrence of allergic reactions. For these allergenic ingredients, no labeling exception is accepted.

Acts

(EU) Regulation no. *1169/2011* of the European Parliament and of the Council of October 25, 2011 on the provision of food information to consumers, amending Regulations (EC) No *1924/2006* and (EC) No *1925/2006* of the European Parliament and of the Council, and repealing Commission Directive *87/250/EEC*, Council Directive *90/496/EEC*, Commission Directive *1999/10/CE*, Directive *2000/13/EC* of the European Parliament and of the Council, Commission Directives *2002/67/EC* and *2008/5/EC* and Commission Regulation (EC) No *608/2004* of the Commission.

This Regulation merges together Directives 2000/13/EC on the *labelling of foodstuffs* and 90/496/EEC on *nutritional labelling* in order to improve the level of consumer information and protection in Europe.

Legislative Regulations

By the political strategy of EU 2007-2013, all the food products in all the manufacturing areas, but traded in the European Community, must be subject to the food consumption laws of Europe.

Regulations
- 178/2002 –general principles concerning food laws
- 258/97 – refers to newly introduced food products
- 1924/2006 – stipulates the nutritional and health provisions/432/2012
- EC 882/2004 – official inspections to check the compliance with the law
- 1925/2006 – additions of vitamins and minerals
- 852/2004 – processing of food products
- 2913/92 – origin of products/country of origin
- The objectives of these regulations aim at protecting consumers' health and at providing proper information

Directives
- 2005/209/EC – misleading publicity and omission of information
- 2000/13/EC – labeling, presentation, publicity
- 90/496/EC – contents and presentation of nutritional information
- 2006/114/EC– publicity

In all the areas of the world, and also according to the number of the persons identified as allergic, there are laws specific to said country.

In USA, the main allergens are: milk, eggs, peanuts, tree nuts (almonds, hazelnuts, cashews, walnuts, etc.), fish, shellfish, soy, and wheat. Food and Drug Administration regulates the food packing manner and the contents of labels.

In Canada, 2% of the population shows risk of anaphylaxis, and the laws refer to: peanuts, almonds, hazelnuts, cashew, walnuts, soy, sesame seeds, wheat, milk, eggs, fish, shellfish and sulfites. The allergens are given priority in the specifications on the label. The labeling must be mandatorily made in

English and French languages. In this country, the Association Quebecoise des Allergies Alimentaires (Quebec Association of Food Allergies) is concerned with the promotion and protection of allergic persons.

In New Zealand, there is a higher risk of allergy to eggs, soy, wheat, milk, peanuts, walnuts, fish and shellfish, and the labeling and packing rules are regulated according to the laws of The Food Standards Australia New Zealand (FSANZ).

Australia is currently represented by Anaphylaxis Australia, which replaced Food Anaphylactic Children Training and Support Association, and which is concerned both with the labeling of food products, and with the prevention of allergies.

The United Kingdom is represented by Anaphylaxis Campaign, and is concerned with the labeling and prevention of allergens. The labeling is regulated by the European laws.

The Netherlands is represented by Netherlands Anafylaxis Network, and the laws refer particularly to the common allergens: peanuts, milk, eggs, wheat, tree nuts (almonds, hazelnut, cashew, walnut, etc.), soy, fish, shellfish, and sesame seed; it is regulated by the European laws.

Italy is represented by Food Allergy Italia. About 6-8% of the population of Italy are allergic to cow's milk, hen's egg, wheat, fish, tree-nut, peanut, and the focus is set on prevention; the laws comply with EU regulations.

In China, the national standards were updated in 2004, according to the Codex Alimentarius Commission; the labeling observes the requested information, without causing confusion, and it is edited both in Chinese, and in English. Therefore, all ingredients including processing aids that constitute part of the food and contain an allergenic substance must be declared in the ingredients list in accordance with paragraph 2(4E) of Schedule 3 to the Food and Drugs (Composition and Labelling) Regulations, Cap. 132W. All the legislative information may be found on the webpage at (http://www.cfs.gov. hk/english/whatsnew/whatsnew_fstr/whatsnew_fstr_13_ins.html)

In Russia – at present, Technical Regulations of the Customs Union were drafted in compliance with the Agreement on Uniform Principles and Rules of Technical Regulation in the Republic of Belarus, the Republic of Kazakhstan and the Russian Federation as of November 18th, 2010. 2. The present Technical Regulations of the Customs Union have been worked out with the purpose of establishing uniform requirements for labeling of food products, obligatory for application and implementation in the unified customs area of the Customs Union and ensuring free circulation of food products released in circulation in the unified customs area of the Customs Union [14].

In the European Community, the labeling of the products complies with the Directive 2000/13/CE) amended with the Directives 2003/89/CE and 2007/68/CE referring to the main allergens included in Codex Alimentarius.

The European Food Safety Authority (EFSA) web site also provides information on food allergen labelling in Europe. The scientific panel responsible for food allergies has for example provided a number of opinions as the scientific basis for the labelling legislation and exemptions from it.

The European Union (EU) improves its regulations concerning the labeling of food products, so that the consumer may get essential, legible and easy to understand information to be able to purchase products knowing well what he purchases. For reasons of public health, the new regulations consolidate the protection against allergens. The ingredients containing peanuts are the ones that are mainly responsible for the occurrence of allergic reactions. For these allergenic ingredients, no labeling exception is accepted.

ACT

(EU) Regulation no. *1169/2011* of the European Parliament and of the Council of October 25, 2011 on the provision of food information to consumers, amending Regulations (EC) No *1924/2006* and (EC) No *1925/2006* of the European Parliament and of the Council, and repealing Commission Directive *87/250/EEC,* Council Directive *90/496/EEC,* Commission Directive *1999/10/CE,* Directive *2000/13/EC* of the European Parliament and of the Council, Commission Directives *2002/67/EC* and *2008/5/EC* and Commission Regulation (EC) No *608/2004* of the Commission.

This Regulation merges together Directives 2000/13/EC on the *labelling of foodstuffs* and 90/496/EEC on *nutritional labelling* in order to improve the level of consumer information and protection in Europe.

This Regulation applies to food business operators at all stages of the food chain. It applies to all foodstuffs intended for the final consumer, including those served by mass caterers, or intended to be delivered to mass caterers.

This Regulation applies without prejudice to the labelling requirements provided for in specific European Union (EU) provisions applicable to particular foodstuffs.

REFERENCES

[1] Sicherer, S.H., Muñoz-Furlong, A., Godbold, J.H., Sampson, H.A., (2010). US prevalence of self-reported peanut, tree nut, and sesame allergy: 11-year follow-up. *J. Allergy Clin. Immunol.* 125(6), 1322-1326.

[2] Boye, J.I., (2012). Food allergies in developing and emerging economies: need for comprehensive data on prevalence rates, *Clinical Translational Allergy.* 2, 25, Online: doi: *10.1186/2045-7022-2-25.*

[3] Leung, T.F., Yung, E., Wong, Y.S., Lam, C.W.K., Wong, G.W.K., (2009). Parent-reported adverse food reactions in Hong Kong Chinese pre-schoolers: epidemiology, clinical spectrum and risk factors. *Pediatr. Allergy Immunol.* 20, 339–346.

[4] Hill, D.J., Hosking, C.S., Zhie, C.Y., Leung, R., Baratwidjaja, K., Iikura, Y., Iyngkaran, N., Gonzalez-Andaya, A., Wah, L.B., Hsieh, K.H., (1997). The frequency of food allergy in Australia and Asia. *Environ. Toxicol. Pharmacol.* 4, 101-110.

[5] Aba-Alkhail, B.A., El-Gamal, F.M.,(2000). Prevalence of food allergy in asthmatic patients. *Saudi Med. J.* 21(1), 81–87.

[6] Westritschnig, K., Sibanda, E., Thomas, W., Auer, H, Aspöck, H., Pittner, G., Vrtala, S., Spitzauer, S., Kraft, D., Valenta, R., (2003). Analysis of the sensitization profile towards allergens in central Africa. *Clin. Exp. Allergy* 33(1), 22–27.

[7] Ouahidi, I., Aarab, L., Dutau, G., (2010). The effect of thermic and acid treatment on the allergenicity of peanut proteins among the population of the region of Fes-Meknes in Morocco. *Rev. Francaise d'Allergol.* 50(1), 15–21.

[8] Obeng, B.B., Amoah, A.S., Larbi, I.A., Yazdanbakhsh, M., van Ree, R., Boakye, D.A., hartgers, F.C., (2011). Food allergy in Ghanaian schoolchildren: data on sensitization and reported food allergy. *Int. Arch. Allergy Immunol.* 155, 63–73.

[9] Levin, M.E., Muloiwa, R., Motala, C.,(2011). Associations between asthma and bronchial hyper-responsiveness with allergy and atopy phenotypes in urban black South African teenagers. *South African Med J.* 101(7), 472–476.

[10] Hossny, E., Gad, G., Shehab, A., El-Haddad, A., (2011). Peanut sensitization in a group of allergic Egyptian children. *Allergy Asthma Clin. Immunol.* 7, 11–17.

[11] Ramos Morín, C.J., Canseco González, C., (1993). Hypersensitivity to common allergens in the central region of Coahuila. *Rev. Alerg. Mex.* 40(6), 150–154.

[12] Ávila Castañón, L., Pérez López, J., Del Río Navarro, B.E., Rosas Vargas, M.A., Lerma Ortiz, L., Sienra Monge, J.J.L., (2002). Food hypersensitivity by skin test in allergic patients at hospital infantil de Mexico Federico Gomez. *Rev. Alerg. Mex.* 49(3), 74–79.

[13] Nabavi, M., Hoseinzadeh, Y., Ghorbani, R., Nabavi, M.,(2010). Prevalence of food allergy in asthmatic children under 18 years of age in semnan-iran in 2007–2008. *Koomesh.*11, 162–169.

[14] Kolchevnikova, O., (2013). Russian Organic Market Continues to Grow. *Russian Federation*, http://gain.fas.usda.gov/

[15] http://www.foodallergy.org/Advocacy/labeling.htmlAllie the Allergic Elephant: A Children's Story of Peanut Allergies" http://www.food allergy.org/Advocacy/labeling.html.

[16] Guidance notes and best practice on allergen and miscellaneous labelling provisions *(July 2008)*; Guidance on allergen management and consumer information *(July 2006);* http://ec.europa.eu/food/food/labeling nutrition/ foodlabelling/index_en.htm.

About the Editors

Maria Pele
University of Agronomic Sciences and Veterinary Medicine
Faculty of Biotechnology
Bucharest, Romania
mpele1950@gmail.com

Carmen Cimpeanu
University of Agronomic Sciences and Veterinary Medicine
Faculty of Biotechnology
Bucharest, Romania
carmencimpeanu@yahoo.com

INDEX